CW00402929

THE GOOD NEWS ABOUT BOOZE

Tony Edwards

Copyright © 2013 Tony Edwards

ISBN 978-0-9566561-4-8

Published by
Premium Publishing
London W12 9RW

First published 2013

Tony Edwards has asserted his right to be identified as the author
of this work in accordance with the Copyright, Designs and
Patents Act 1988.

All rights reserved. No part of this publication may be
reproduced, stored in a retrieval system, or transmitted in any
form or by any means, electronic, mechanical, photocopying or
otherwise without the prior permission of the author.

A CIP record of this book is available from the British Library.

Cover design by Lewis Kokoc
Grams graphics by Robert Norman-Reade

Typesetting, design and layout by
amandahelm@helm-information.co.uk

For Debs,
my rock and pal through thick and thin.
Cheers, darling!

Contents

Acknowledgements

As with most modern in-depth writing about medicine, this book would not have been possible without the generosity of 1. the American taxpayer for PubMed, the online medical database, and 2. Larry Page and Sergey Brin for Google Scholar, the almost omniscient 21st c. Library of Alexandria, whose treasures are accessible even from rural England within seconds. The magnificent librarians at the Royal Society of Medicine provided unlimited access to the full texts of published papers. My Psychology graduate daughter Charlotte helped collate the references and my Economics undergraduate son Joe constructed the graphs. Thanks also to mathematician and health author Zoe Harcombe for helping me interpret the more recondite statistics in some individual studies, and to Professors Caroline Taylor and Karol Sikora for valuable comments on the MS – plus of course huge gratitude to the latter for generously offering to write the Foreword. However, it goes without saying that I am solely responsible for the book's contents and the views expressed.

Author's Note

This book attempts to distil about half a million scientific papers on alcohol and health. In reporting the studies' findings, it occasionally draws inferences about their practical import for the individual. However, the book is essentially a reportage, and is not intended as health advice. The information and opinions provided here are believed to be accurate and sound and are based on the best judgments of the author. However, readers should make their own enquiries and consult knowledgeable health professionals before acting upon anything they read in this book.

Neither the author nor the publisher can be held responsible nor liable for any loss or claim arising from the use, or misuse, of the information in this book.

The Author

Tony Edwards is a former BBC tv science producer, now writer on science and medicine. Most of his career was spent with *Horizon* and *QED*, where six ($\approx10\%$) of his programmes received international awards, including the British Medical Association's "Medicine in the Media" – the BMA's top media gong. An ischemic stroke in his 50s put paid to tv production, whereupon he took up the pen, initially writing on technology, but latterly on medicine, for a wide variety of publications. He is married to broadcaster Debbie Rix, now communications consultant and writer (of fiction). They have two children and live in rural Kent.

Foreword

Professor Karol Sikora

Consultant Oncologist,
Dean of Britain's first independent Medical School
at the University of Buckingham

Booze kills. Booze ruins lives, destroys families, ends successful careers, causes untold physical and mental illness and has a huge adverse impact on society. If you have the misfortune to be in a hospital Emergency Room late on a Saturday night you will see unbelievable scenes of social degradation caused by alcohol. The cost in human, monetary and societal terms is just staggering. So why is a doctor who specialises in cancer treatment writing a Foreword for a book like this? After all, the whole healthcare system continuously bombards us with the evils of drink. How can there be any good news at all?

Science is all about evidence. Observational and experimental data are collected, assessed, dissected, re-examined and conclusions drawn in a fair and unbiased way. Often the end results do not fit our preconceived notions. That's the excitement of science – it can change our perception of the world around us. The world is not flat, matter and energy are inter-convertible, the atom can be split and cells divide by intricate chemical processes within their DNA. It's all based on good evidence.

What science writer Tony Edwards has done here is to gather up all the evidence on alcohol's good side (plus some of its bad side) in one place. He's painstakingly gone through reams of often extremely dull text published in impenetrable medical journals. He's taken the data and processed it in a very understandable way. And you will find he has a great, if a little quirky, sense of humour which makes it a far better read than a dry old textbook. Whether you're teetotal, an occasional pint person or an avid wine buff, the book will be of considerable interest.

Health education systems globally tend to simplify their messages. There is no room for doubt. They have to get through clearly to as many people as possible of different educational backgrounds. Unknowns get taken over by evangelical half-truths. The complex becomes simple. Were you aware that even the safe number of units of alcohol we can drink was originally based on a back of an envelope calculation by a committee of the great and the good back in the late 1980s ? Each country has its own views - and that's precisely why there is no internationally agreed maximum safe daily intake. Bias confounds all the messages. Everybody is selling you a line. Governments want you to drink less, as they don't want to spend huge amounts on the social disorder alcohol can cause, medical charities want your donations, so they plug the message that alcohol's bad news, making you feel they care about your health, our NHS doesn't really want you to use its services, and politicians just want your vote so they can go to the bar in the House of Commons – well at least some of them.

When I was a young house physician (the lowest rank of junior doctor) in a famous London teaching hospital as recently as the 1970s, it was standard practice to prescribe sherry, beer, and even whisky and brandy to patients as a "tonic" with their evening meal. We wrote it on the prescription sheet at the end of the bed alongside the antibiotics, immunosuppressants, heart drugs and pain killers. At first I didn't know the dose, so I would write "15ml sherry" … until one nice elderly lady very politely told me she usually got a much larger glass. It was my first example of what would now be called a fully engaged patient giving 360 degree feedback. However, before you book yourself into the local hospital, I am sorry to tell you that those days are long gone, because alcohol is now thought to be dangerous and even "evil". But how can booze be such bad thing if we were encouraged to prescribe it as a drug on the NHS not so very long ago?

Perhaps the most surprising feature of this book is the evidence of obvious benefit from alcohol. As you read on you'll become familiar with the J-curve. If you don't drink at all, you have a defined risk of developing all sorts of medical problems in your heart, joints, brain, blood sugar levels, and kidneys – indeed all round your body. As you begin to drink there seems to be evidence of benefit. As you drink more, that gradually disappears and the damaging effects kick in ... and eventually go above the non-drinking baseline. This creates a health graph resembling the letter J. And most surprisingly of all, how long you will live – your longevity – follows the same J-shaped curve.

Interestingly, different sources of alcohol have different good effects. I am glad to say that there seems reasonable evidence that my own favourite tipple – red wine – seems to have a powerful beneficial effect at the sort of doses I imbibe.

Clearly much more research is needed in this fascinating area. From pharmacology to sociology there is a dearth of meaningful research. New protective mechanisms need to be discovered and new drugs developed to mimic the beneficial effects on the body. Understanding why alcohol leads to addiction in certain people is absolutely critical to the prevention of alcoholism and the downward spiral that it can cause. But simply suppressing the truth and creating confusion in the name of a nanny state is not the way forward.

Of course this book will be labelled as 'controversial'. But its value is that it could lead to a much better understanding of all the complex issues involved. Nothing is necessarily what it seems. Here you have the data you need to help you make your own decision. Yes, drink kills, but it can also have a positive effect on our physical, mental and spiritual wellbeing. You have to come to your own conclusion. My advice is to stay as low as you can on the letter J.

Professor Karol Sikora MA, MB. BChir, PhD, FRCR, FRCP, FFPM

Preface

Imagine this.

Joe Bloggs goes to his GP. "My hands hurt, I get a bit of a pain in my chest sometimes, and I'm beginning to forget things", he complains. The doctor examines him and says: "You've got a touch of arthritis, possibly mild heart disease, and you may be in the first stages of dementia. How much are you drinking?" "Never touch a drop, doc", says Joe proudly. "Ah, that explains it," says the GP, wagging an admonishing finger. "Here's a prescription for red wine – a quarter of a litre a day." "Don't like red wine", splutters the astonished patient. "White wine, Mr Bloggs?" "Don't like wine at all doc, or really any alcohol." "Pity", says the doctor. "In which case, I'll have to give you a prescription for vodka. Drink a double measure every day before or after your evening meal; take the taste away with fruit juice if you like, but make sure you drink it."

Ridiculous? Absurd? A story in the *Bumper Book of Jokes for Alcoholics*? Absolutely not.

Let me tell you this: if GPs fail to recommend alcohol to at least some of their patients, they should be had up for medical negligence. Only joking, but that's the logical conclusion from a mass of scientific research data, the salient bits of which are in this book.

I am well aware that a book which reveals evidence of alcohol's health benefits will not be welcomed by the medical establishment, and that its author will be accused of bias, ignorance, stupidity, trying to justify his own drinking habits, being in the pay of the drinks industry, etc etc.

But I can assure you that this book is more objective about the medical evidence on alcohol and health than anything the vast majority of you will have heard or read before. After months of in-depth research, I have discovered that almost everything that is promulgated about alcohol and health is one-sided propaganda in what appears to be a kind of medical prohibitionist war against alcohol. The fact that we find my GP fantasy so damn silly is a tribute to its success.

I came to write about alcohol only by accident while doing research for an article on calories and weight gain in early 2012. To my surprise I discovered that the clinical data show that alcohol, although laden with calories, does not put on weight. That's odd, I thought; I wonder what else is odd about alcohol … and the more I delved into the evidence, the odder the picture became. Again to my surprise, I found myself confronted with findings that any pharmaceutical company would have been uncorking the champagne over: clear, repeated evidence of substantial health benefits from alcohol.

And yet the endlessly repeated public message is that alcohol is Bad News. This is of course true: alcohol can indeed be harmful … but most of the time it isn't, and can actually be beneficial. So it's a complex picture. But to show only one side of the picture, as the medical authorities overwhelmingly do, is Bad Medicine because it prevents people making sensible decisions about healthy lifestyle choices. This book may help.

It's been written therefore more as a medical reference book for the layman (and perhaps even GPs!) than a fluffy narrative about Bordeaux-swilling French centenarians, beaming German brewmasters, or the personal lives of the world's top alcohol experts … just their scientific research. So it's a bit of a slog through a litany of (fully referenced) evidence,* leavened by occasional light-hearted asides, common-sense comments, and forays into the first person – which should not, however, be taken to imply that you'll be reading a personal view.

This book is what it says on the tin: a sober, evidence-based synthesis of the surprisingly Good News About Booze.

Tony Edwards   *October 2013*

---

* Although the book refers to data derived from animals, this does not imply endorsement of such research methods – in this field particularly.

1

Introduction

Doctors used to nag us about smoking, but now that politicians have got the message about tobacco, it's alcohol that's been put in the naughty corner. And doctors can get quite moralistic about it. A few years ago, the Royal College of Physicians in Britain produced a report on alcohol with the bizarre title: "Alcohol – a great and growing Evil".[1] Why bizarre? Is evil really a medical adjective? "A great and growing problem", maybe, but only the religious professions are licensed to talk of evil, surely – not medics.

That "evil" RCP report came out in 1987, but every few years since then, we've been subjected to another tongue-lashing from one set of medical prelates or another: no less than two reports in 1995, another in 2001, and one in 2010:[2–5]

And that's not counting sporadic sermons from the Department of Health, the National Audit Office, the Heart Foundation, Cancer Research UK, and the Uncle Tom Cobley Association. Not to mention occasional jihads from such bodies as the awkwardly named Change4Life, started in 2012. As an example of the propaganda, here's part of one of their press releases:

> Drinking too much is a major public health issue. This campaign highlights how easy it can be to use a glass of wine or beer to unwind at the end of a busy day, but these drinks stack up and can increase your risk of high blood pressure, cancer or liver disease.

The problem with this statement is this. Yes, alcohol can indeed have all those scary-sounding effects, but quite a lot of the time these are outweighed by booze's benefits, as the scientific evidence outlined in this book will show. Why didn't Change4Life's campaign managers tell you that

? Because they'd rather you got the message that "drinking too much is a major public health issue".

How much is "too much"?

It wasn't until the 1987 Royal College of Physicians report that doctors decided they perhaps ought to work out how dangerous boozing actually was. After all, if they wanted to call it "evil" they needed some justification. So they set up a committee of experts chaired by the then Editor of the BMJ, Dr Richard Smith, in order to recommend maximum drinking limits.

However, the whole exercise was somewhat haphazard, as Dr Smith admitted 25 years later: "I remember the debate when the epidemiologist said it was impossible to set limits because the evidence was poor; but we agreed that it was better to offer some advice rather than none, and that it needed to be simple."[6]

The figures they arrived at were 21 "units" a week for men and 14 for women, with one unit being 8 grams of alcohol – roughly equal to a measure of spirits, half a pint of beer or a tenth of a bottle of wine. Interviewed about five years later by a Times journalist, Dr Smith confessed that the figures "were plucked out of the air. They were not based on any firm evidence at all. It was a sort of intelligent guess by a committee."[7]

Dr Smith is aware his frankness hasn't exactly endeared him to his fellow medics, but he was right. The limits were indeed pretty arbitrary, and based on precious little scientific evidence. However, they have remained exactly the same ever since.

An indication of just how plucked out of the air the UK figures really are comes from the fact that no two countries' medical authorities agree on what's a maximum safe limit. While (for men) in the UK it's 32 grams of alcohol a day, in Australia it's 40 grams, in Portugal 37 grams, and in Sweden 20.[8]

In fact, twelve countries recommend lower limits than the UK for women, fifteen countries lower limits for men, and six countries recommend higher limits for both men and women than in the UK. Even more absurdly, there are disagreements between one country's own "authorities". For example, in the USA, the National Institute of Alcohol Abuse & Alcoholism says the upper safe limit is 56 grams a day, but the Department of Health thinks it's 28. France is even crazier: its Ministry of Health says the maximum is 20 grams a day, but its Academy of Medicine says "non, c'est 60".

To make matters worse, countries' official bodies don't use understandable measures like grams or ounces of alcohol, but what they call "units" or "drinks". That might be OK if everyone could agree on what these terms actually stand for. But they can't. For example, while in the UK one "unit" equals 8 grams of alcohol, in the USA it's 14 grams, in Denmark 12, and in Japan 19.5. Helpfully, there is an "international unit" which is 10 grams, but unhelpfully many countries ignore it.

There's a body called ICAP (International Center for Alcohol Policies) which sounds as though it ought to oversee international alcohol standards, but it's in fact toothless. All it can do is bleat about the current shambles:

> The way in which the concept of a standard drink is currently implemented within an international setting is less than optimal. The manner in which standard drinks are applied can be confusing. International comparisons are made difficult by a wide range of definitions. This disparity is often not taken into consideration when information on drinking guidelines from different countries, often given in terms of standard drinks or units, is interpreted and compared.[9]

ICAP wrote that in 1998, but since then nothing's happened. Alcohol units and guidelines are still as "confusing" as ever.

The temptation to observe that medics couldn't organise the proverbial piss-up in a brewery is overwhelming*.

One consequence of this "drinks/units" shambles is that it can be difficult for medical researchers to compare data

---
*   "The only way to get rid of a temptation is to yield to it", Oscar Wilde.

across national boundaries – a problem which it's been suggested accounts for some of the discrepancies in the research findings. It also makes it a pain for science writers such as myself, because many researchers report their findings only in terms of "units" or "drinks", rather than grams of alcohol.

So, when assessing and reporting the medical findings in this book, I have followed the procedure used by all the professional research analysts: to convert the "drink/units" measures into grams according to the national figures of the particular research group.

Inside the back and front covers, you'll find two ways of showing the average alcohol content of standard drinks, so you can refer to them as you read.

Now, let's take a long look at the evidence. However, before embarking on the Good News, it would be irresponsible not to confront the Bad News. But don't despair: it's only one chapter, and it's got a fair sprinkling of Good News buried within it.

Let me reiterate the health warning before the Preface, however.

Nothing in this book should be interpreted as a health recommendation. Like any individual newspaper journalist's assessment of the results of a pharmaceutical drug trial, for example, the author merely sets out his assessments of the results of medical investigations into alcohol. If readers wish to act on any of the information in the book, they are urged to make their own assessments of the medical evidence (via PubMed or similar), or obtain informed advice before doing so.

2

The Bad News

The ostensible reason why our medical masters are so down on the drink is because of their apparent concern for our health. And my goodness, how keen they are to finger-wag at us. Seemingly not a month is allowed to pass without some media-trained academic being paraded in front of the press, armed with the shock results of his or her latest scare-mongering study.

One of the medics' constantly reiterated campaigns has been to attack the bourgeoisie for the huge amount their drinking is apparently costing health services.

"Baby boomers are draining NHS resources through alcohol misuse" said a press release in October 2012, claiming that the 55–74 age group is costing the British taxpayer nearly £2 billion a year. Written by a UK charity called Alcohol Concern, it went on:

> It is the common perception that young people are responsible for the increasing cost of alcohol misuse, but our findings show that in reality this is not the case. It is the middle-aged, and often middle class drinker, regularly drinking above recommended limits, who are actually requiring complex and expensive NHS care.[1]

The NHS agrees that adult drinkers are wrecking their health, with their own website[2] claiming that:

> There are many long-term health risks associated with alcohol misuse. They include:
> high blood pressure (hypertension)
> stroke
> heart disease
> pancreatitis
> liver disease
> liver cancer

cancer of the mouth
head and neck cancer
breast cancer
bowel cancer
dementia
sexual problems, such as impotence or premature ejaculation

That's a typical litany of health conditions routinely laid at alcohol's door ... and obediently trotted out in the media, so they'll be pretty familiar to you.

But let's examine them closely, and see how true they really are, or whether the statements are being "economical with the actualité" (a franglais euphemism coined by British MP Alan Clark – perhaps appropriately, the only Cabinet minister to have been accused of giving a drunken speech in Parliament!)

Read on.

The Big C

Let's start with cancer, the bogeyman disease we fear most and whose incidence is rising inexorably. Could alcohol be responsible? That's a question medics have spent years and millions of pounds and dollars trying to answer, obviously hoping the answer is yes.

By 2007, researchers had done more than 500 medical studies on the connection between alcohol and cancers of all types, and that year the World Cancer Research Fund decided to pool the studies' findings to see how they panned out. Claimed to be "the most comprehensive report ever produced on the links between lifestyle and cancer risk" and "the best advice available anywhere in the world on how to reduce cancer risk", the WCRF Report was a massive undertaking, in which over 200 doctors round the world ploughed their way through billions of bits of data. At the time of writing, that Report remains the supreme source of data on alcohol and cancer.[3]

So what do WRCF say about it?

Let's start with their conclusion. "From the point of view of cancer prevention, the best level of alcohol consumption is zero." Sounds authoritative, final and stark – and scary. But if you examine the details of the Report, you'll get a picture that's rather more nuanced.

Let's look at the detailed evidence, cancer type by cancer type.

Bowel Cancer

This cancer of the colon (large intestine) is the third most common cancer, accounting for about 10% of all cancers worldwide. What does the WCRF report say about booze's role in all this?

> The evidence that consumption of more than 30 g/day of ethanol from alcoholic drinks is a cause of colorectal cancer in men is convincing, and probably also in women.

Plain language: a chap's bowels should be OK cancer-wise if he drinks less than 30 grams of alcohol[*] (about a third of a bottle of wine or 1½ pints of beer) a day; above that there will be a risk … but possibly not for ladies.[†]

However, if you burrow into the evidence as a whole, the alcohol/bowel cancer connection is rather confused, exposing disagreements between different research teams. For example, one huge UK-based study in 2010 analysed the medical data from over 150,000 British drinkers and non-drinkers, and could find no "statistically significant" (i.e. meaningful) connection between alcohol and bowel cancer whatever – however much anyone drank.[4]

---

[*] I am aware that grams are an unusual measure of alcohol content, but you're going to have to get used to them, as they're used throughout the book. Rather than having constantly to explain what they mean in everyday terms, there are two styles of gram content illustrations on the last two pages of the book, so you can refer to them as you read.

[†] An updated 2010 Report modified this conclusion by claiming that even small amounts of alcohol have some bowel cancer risk; however, much of the new data came from studies on Asians (therefore of a special genetic type – see Chapter 10), and also was not statistically significant .

On the other hand, researchers across the English Channel disagree, because they think that there is booze/bowel cancer connection, having discovered that drinkers of more than 60 grams of alcohol a day roughly double their risk of the disease. [5]

Sounds like serious Bad News ... but is it?

Not really. Twice the risk is no big deal when you compare it to the risk of lung cancer and smoking, for example, which is about 25-fold.

Also, as far as bowel cancer is concerned, drinking appears to be no more dangerous than eating red or processed meat. Studies show that both have much the same effect on cancer risk.[6]

And when have you ever heard medics fulminating against meat-eaters or encouraging us all to become vegetarians?

You're right: never.

In fact, most experts think the alcohol/bowel cancer risk is pretty small beer. For example, a massive international study done by Harvard University found that "alcohol intake correlates with a modest relative elevation in colon cancer rate, mainly at the highest levels of alcohol intake"[7] – in plain language, drinkers don't have much of a risk of bowel cancer, and even heavy drinkers aren't greatly affected.

Indeed, there's some evidence that one type of alcohol may actually protect against the cancer.

In 2009 Cambridge University researchers reported the results of an 11 year long study of almost 25,000 folk in Norfolk, tracking their alcohol intake and bowel cancer incidence. The extraordinary connection they found was that drinking wine actually seemed to reduce the risk of the cancer. Here's their final quote: "Daily consumption of more than 8 grams of wine appeared inversely related to colorectal cancer risk (HR: 0.61)". Translated into English, that means Norfolk wine drinkers have almost half the risk of bowel cancer of non-drinkers [8].

Lest you imagine that study was a freak East Anglian result, two American surveys have also found a similar protective effect from wine, and to a lesser extent, even from alcohol itself at low doses [9] [10]. But it's fair to say, that's not a universal finding.

Nevertheless, the totality of the evidence suggests that your bowel has nothing too much to fear from alcohol, and indeed possibly something to gain if you choose your tipple wisely.

Liver Cancer

If there's one organ that doctors tell drinkers that alcohol is bad for, it's the liver. It causes both liver cancer as well as cirrhosis.

Certainly, it's not unreasonable to suppose that the liver might be badly affected by alcohol: after all, alcohol is a toxin, and the liver is where all poisons – from pesticides to potatoes[*] – get detoxified.

So, few of us will be surprised by the idea that alcohol and livers don't mix. That's what doctors tell us anyway. But what does the evidence really say? Once again, it turns out that we're only given a partial view of the true picture.

The facts are these: yes, alcohol almost certainly causes liver cancer (which they tell you), but for most drinkers it almost certainly doesn't (which of course they don't).

Let's tunnel into the mountain of data assembled by the WCRF Report, which looked at a couple of dozen studies specifically investigating the liver cancer/alcohol link. To judge from the propaganda message about the issue, you'd think the evidence would be clear-cut, with drinkers being found to drop like flies from liver cancer. Not a bit of it. Summarising the studies, the Report had to admit (in small print) that the data had:

> high heterogeneity [in which] a dose-response relationship
> is apparent from case-control but not cohort data.

---

[*]   Potatoes contain a poison which, if you were to eat a small sackful of spuds, could kill you.

In plain language: the findings of these studies are extremely inconsistent; furthermore, there is no clear pattern linking increasing alcohol intake with increased liver cancer.

The best the Report felt able to conclude was that "alcohol is a probable cause of liver cancer" – "probable" ... hardly a ringing condemnation.

In any case, even assuming a probable connection, one again needs to ask: how much extra risk of liver cancer do drinkers actually run?

It's not easy to come up with a figure – not least because roughly half the liver cancer studies are 'not statistically significant'. This fact alone suggests that the alcohol/liver cancer connection is pretty weak. However, taking the data at face value, the extra risk appears to no greater than for bowel cancer. Also, the type of alcohol could be important: wine may be completely innocent – although the evidence is only suggestive at present.[11] [12]

Incidentally, in animal experiments, when researchers tested alcohol on mice already injected with a poison designed to cause liver cancer, they found alcohol "unexpectedly" prevented cancer formation.[13] They had to do all sorts of nasty things to the animals before their livers conformed to the prevailing theory.

Liver Cirrhosis
When livers and alcohol mentioned, it's cirrhosis that people mostly think of; because cirrhosis can be a precursor of cancer, I'll deal with it here.

Cirrhosis of the liver is the No. 1 hazard medical pro-hibitionists like to scare us with. For example, in a 2012 BBC tv programme on alcoholism,[14] pathologists excised whole cirrhotic livers from dead alcoholics and sternly waved them in front of the camera – as in some totemic voodoo ritual. However, once again, doctors may be guilty of over-egging the pudding.

The catch-all term for liver problems thought to be caused by alcohol is Alcohol Liver Disease (ALD). And the facts are that ALD is not nearly as widespread as doctors like to make out.

Here's the evidence.

In the 1980s Danish researchers decided to track the health of more than 13000 people over a 12-year period, specifically looking for a connection between alcohol and ALD.[15] As expected, they found that, above an intake of about 35 grams a day, there was indeed a risk of ALD. But, crucially, this risk only applied to a relatively few people. Fully 93% of the drinkers had no sign of cirrhosis whatever, even at alcohol intakes above 120 grams a day.

A previous study by another Danish research group came up with similar findings.[16] 258 initially healthy male drinkers were tracked for 13 years to see how many developed ALD. The men were chosen specifically because they were all "alcohol abusing" ... and yet fewer than 7% of them developed cirrhosis.

Italian doctors found very much the same thing in a celebrated study called "Dionysos" in 1997.[17] This was an intensive long-term study of the inhabitants of two towns in northern Italy. Evidently, some of these 7000 Italian townsfolk were pretty heavy drinkers, with over a hundred of them downing the equivalent of more than a bottle and a half of wine a day – and yet the vast majority of these heavy boozers had no ALD symptoms at all. "Even at an intake of over 120 grams of alcohol a day, the percentage of subjects with alcohol-induced liver damage was relatively low – 13.5%", the researchers reported. At lower intakes, they also found puzzlingly low levels of ALD. Above an intake of 30 grams a day, "only 5.5% of the individuals showed signs of liver damage, and 'pure' alcoholic cirrhosis in 2.2%", they said.

Liver disease is also rare even in the most severe alcoholics, according to researchers in Sweden – where alcoholism is rife. A large study in 2008 reported finding that only 1 in 5 serious alcoholics get cirrhosis, and that the

11

ones who do aren't necessarily the heaviest drinkers.[18]

Why do so few drinkers get ALD? Some experts believe the answer lies in people's genetic make-up.

A group of Italian geneticists made a special study of the heavy drinkers in the Dionysos population, and found that cirrhosis tended to occur in the people who had particularly unusual variants of the two genes responsible for detoxifying alcohol in the liver.[19] These genetic variants "are very low in Caucasians", they acknowledged. Liver experts in Finland have found very much the same.[20]

So, the evidence is now pretty clear that if you're unlucky enough to have the wrong genes, you might get ALD almost no matter how little you drink. With the right genes, however, you'll probably never get liver disease. Fortunately, the vast majority of us seem to have the right genes, which explains why the vast majority of drinkers don't get liver disease.*

For the few genetic unfortunates, however, there are two possible remedies: drink lots of coffee[21] and take Vitamin B supplements.[22] Both significantly reduce the risk of ALD, but no-one tells you any of this.

What doctors also don't tell you is that some kinds of liver disease might actually be prevented by alcohol – for example, a condition called Fatty Liver Disease (steatohepatatis).

Astonishingly, a huge USA-wide survey in 2012 found that alcohol is of real benefit for this fairly common liver problem.[23] "Our study showed that people with modest alcohol intake – up to 36 grams of alcohol daily – had half the risk of developing steatohepatitis than people who drank no alcohol," reported lead author Professor Jeffrey Schwimmer of UC San Diego. What makes this finding even more extraordinary is that steatohepatitis is a forerunner of both cirrhosis and liver cancer.

So we now have two cogent explanations for why so few drinkers have liver problems: first, genetics, and second, alcohol's wholly surprising preventive effect at an intake of up to 36 grams a day.

---

*   See chapter 10 for more about genes.

There's a massive "on the other hand" postscript, however. One group of drinkers have a huge (up to a 100-fold) risk of ALD: people already suffering from liver disease, in particular Hepatitis C.[24] The disease is mainly confined to intravenous drug users and people with HIV.

Head, Neck and Mouth Cancers
That's what the NHS calls them, rather confusingly. Their correct medical terms are: cancers of the larynx, oesophagus and oral cavity, ie cancers of the parts of the body alcohol hits first: mouth, throat and gullet. You may have seen the almost unrecognisable pictures of journalist Christopher Hitchens as he underwent chemotherapy – ultimately futilely – for oesophageal cancer in 2011. He had been a very heavy drinker and smoker.

Of all the cancers, these three are far and away the most obviously caused by alcohol. However, although the evidence is strong, it's not nearly as clear-cut as that linking smoking and lung cancer, for example, as there's quite a lot of heterogeneity and inconsistency between the various studies. But what's impressive is that there's a fairly consistent dose-response effect. Also, of all the claimed alcohol-related cancers, these three seem to have the most likely causation: localised damage to the tissues – possibly to do with DNA (see later in this chapter).

However, the WCRF Report admits that the actual risk of these cancers is not huge. Averaging out the data, it says if you imbibe 3 US "drinks" per day (that's about 42 grams) you'll only double the risk – pretty insignificant, especially as the diseases themselves are so rare.

It's the combination with smoking that's the real killer, because the risk increases dramatically if you smoke.[25]

But it's not all Bad News, because once again there's some bizarre evidence that alcohol may actually help reduce the risk of some of these cancers. Two separate research teams in the USA and Australia[26][27] have investigated the incidence of a condition called Barrett's Esophagus, and found that wine and beer drinkers have less risk of the disease than non-drinkers. Why is this bizarre? Because Barrett's Esophagus is the main precursor of oesophageal cancer, of which alcohol is believed to be a major cause.

However, that paradox is solved by the fact that there are two types of oesophageal cancer. The 'squamous cancer' type is pretty clearly caused by alcohol,[28] while the other 'adenocarcinoma' type isn't … and that's the one which is becoming a growing problem, possibly due to increasing obesity.[29]

Breast Cancer
Highly emotive, of course, and therefore one that our prohibitionist authorities like to harp on about. For example, Cancer Research UK warns of the "strong evidence that drinking even small amounts of alcohol increases the risk of breast cancer".

Once again, let's test that statement against the actual evidence.

The WCRF Report examined over 100 separate studies investigating the alcohol/breast cancer link, and found what it called "high heterogeneity" – a jargon term meaning the results were all over the place. So, depending on which study you chose, you could be frightened out of your wits by reading that a gin and tonic might trigger major breast cancer, or instantly organise a boozy girls night out, having read that a quarter of a bottle of wine a day would prevent it.

What's more, many of these studies were what medical statisticians call "non-significant", i.e. they could have been chance results. Given such messy data, common-sense suggests that there probably isn't much of a connection between alcohol and breast cancer, according to at least some experts. "Studies can have conflicting results mainly because the association between alcohol and breast cancer is rather weak", says Dr Curtis Ellison, Professor of Medicine

& Public Health at Boston University School of Medicine. The prestigious US Government's National Institute of Alcohol Abuse and Alcoholism (NIAAA) agrees, pointing out "the inconsistency and weakness of the epidemiologic findings" with breast cancer[30] and the "lack of understanding of how and when alcohol consumption impacts breast cancer risk".[31]

Since the publication of the WCRF report, however, there have been a few more studies which tend to be more positive about the breast cancer/alcohol link.

Nevertheless, the more recent investigations are still pretty contradictory. For example, a Harvard study shows a "small increase in risk" after drinking tiny amounts of alcohol,[32] while another one conducted down the coast in New York, although agreeing low intakes are associated with a "modest" increase in risk, found intakes above 30 grams perfectly safe.[33]

A 2007 Danish paper further muddies the waters.[34] Headed by Professor Morten Grønbaek, one of the world's top alcohol researchers, the study followed nearly 18,000 nurses for 8 years; all were free of cancer at the start, and most of them were drinkers – some rather heavy ones, too. The results were astonishing, completely contradicting the claim of there being "strong evidence that drinking even small amounts of alcohol increases the risk of breast cancer". For example, Grønbaek found that the nurses who drank small amounts of alcohol actually reduced their breast cancer risk compared to their teetotal colleagues – a protection that persisted up to an intake of 24 grams of alcohol a day. Above that, the cancer risk increased, but not at all consistently. See overleaf for a graph of Grønbaek's results.

As you can see, the Danish nurses' breast cancer risk *decreased* at intakes up to 24 grams a day,* rose steeply to 100% (i.e. double the risk) at intakes of 36–46 grams a day,

---

* A similar reduction in breast cancer risk at low alcohol intake levels was observed in Britain's "Million Women" Study in 2009, but that fact was buried in the small print of the paper.

but fell back to 25% at higher intakes still. If there's really a breast cancer/alcohol connection, those reductions at both low and high doses don't make sense.

Grønbaek found similarly paradoxical results with binge drinking – defined by him as over 60 grams a day. The nurses who drank at those levels had a 45% increase in risk, but those who drank even more (bingeing on 72 grams a day) had 18% less risk of breast cancer than teetotallers. That's bonkers.

Critics may well say that these kinds of strange results at high intakes may have been flukes, possibly to do with the relatively small numbers of heavy female drinkers, but as Grønbaek points out, three other studies have come up with similar results.[35] [36] [37]

There's some equally strange breast cancer data with alcoholics. A huge 30-year study on over 36,000 Swedish female alcoholics found that "contrary to expectation" these by definition exceptionally heavy drinkers had only a "small 15% increase in breast cancer risk compared to the general female population".[38] This was no flash in the pan study either. It was a collaboration between experts at two pinnacle institutions: Harvard and the Karolinska Institute, who admit their findings are a 'paradox'. "Our data challenge a monotonic causal association between alcohol and breast cancer," they say ruefully.

Another surprise is that women already diagnosed with breast cancer have been found slightly to reduce their risk of dying if they drink.[39]

Similarly, there's some heart-warming medical science for female *bon viveurs* in a 2008 French study on women whose favourite tipple was red wine.[40] It showed that those who drank about a sixth of a bottle of wine a day *halved their risk* of breast cancer. Above that intake, the benefit was found to fall away, but without raising the cancer risk above the teetotal level.

We'll take a long look at wine in Chapter 12.

However, countering all this inconsistent evidence are

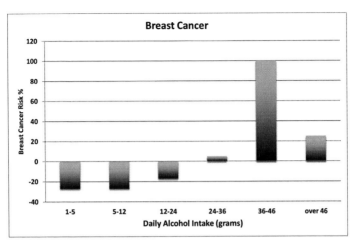

Derived from: Grønbaek M et al. *Eur J Public Health* (2007) 17 (6): 624–629. Alcohol drinking, consumption patterns and breast cancer among Danish nurses: a cohort study.

the results of a massive European-wide survey published in 2011.[41] It involved over 250,000 women, and came to the conclusion that between 2% and 8% of breast cancer cases could be "attributable to alcohol". That's a significant number, but the researchers had to admit one strong caveat: "if we assume causality".

That "causality" problem bedevils much of the alcohol/ cancer issue, i.e. even if there is an apparent connection between alcohol intake and cancer rates, how can you be sure that one actually causes the other? For example, if bird-watchers noticed an increase in stork numbers one year and there was a corresponding increase in the human birth rate, could you conclude storks are somehow connected with births? We'll come back to the causality issue at the end of this chapter.

To discover if alcohol really causes breast cancer, you'd need to do a controlled experiment. Ideally you should put two groups of identical women in identical circumstances and give one group alcoholic drinks and the other group fake alcoholic drinks … and then monitor them for at least a decade – for lots of reasons, clearly impossible.

But there is a fall-back solution which is almost as good: if you can't experiment on women, use mice instead.

Fortunately for scientific researchers (but not of course for the animals), drug companies have developed strains of mice which are particularly prone to breast cancer – mainly for the purpose of testing anti-cancer drugs.

In 1992, pharmacologists at the University of Florida gave different doses of alcohol to some of these mice in controlled laboratory conditions, and compared them with identical mice given simply water.[42] The results were clear-cut, and a serious blow to the alcohol/breast cancer advocates. This is what happened to the mice … nothing:

> Despite administration of ethanol to isocalorically fed C3H/Ou mice for 65 weeks by three different methods, mammary tumor development was not enhanced.

In other words, alcohol had zero effect on the mice's breast cancer development, despite them a. having been forced to drink alcohol every day for over a year, and b. being pre-programmed to get breast cancer.

So is that the end of it? Can we now conclude that the alcohol/breast cancer connection really may be spurious? No. Biology is not as cut and dried as 'hard' sciences like physics.

For in 2000, Japanese animal researchers tested alcohol on a different strain of genetically engineered mice, and found that 45% of them got breast cancer.[43] However, the study was later criticised[44] for using 'the wrong kind of mice' (my expression), but that hasn't stopped it being widely used as evidence in favour of the alcohol/breast cancer link.

And … er, that's it.

The plain fact is that, apart from that study, no animal studies have ever confirmed the alcohol/breast cancer link, except by doing unpleasant things to the animals beforehand – a fact acknowledged in an authoritative report in 2012.[45]

For example, in 2010, University of Texas nutritionists, puzzled that alcohol didn't seem to produce breast cancer in mice, had to inject the animals with actual breast cancer cells before they could get the "model" to work.[46] Lo and behold, they found that all the mice developed breast cancer, but the ones given alcohol got larger tumours. Women don't get breast cancer by having cancer cells injected into them, of course.

What conclusions can be drawn from these conflicting animal studies? The same conclusion as from the human studies ... that the whole evidence base for the breast cancer/alcohol link seems to be a mess.

In August 2012, Professor Harvey Finkel of Boston University, cancer expert and member of the International Scientific Forum on Alcohol Research, summed it up like this: "The role of alcohol in the genesis of breast cancer has continued to be confusing, even conflicted," he says.[47]

But let's err on the side of caution, put aside the contradictions in the evidence, and allow for a genuine alcohol/breast cancer link. What is the most solid evidence the hawks have come up with?

To date, one of the biggest investigations* was done by experts at various universities (including Harvard) in the 1980/90s. It was an 11-year study involving a total of 322,647 women in the USA, Canada, Sweden and Holland.[48] The researchers found that drinking between 30 and 60 grams of alcohol a day was associated with a 41% increase in breast cancer risk. Sounds scary ... until one does the maths. First, 41% is less than half double the extra risk – small potatoes compared to a 25 times extra lung cancer risk from smoking, for example. Second, 41% is a "Relative Risk" not an "Absolute Risk".

Why is that an important difference?

The sad fact is that quite a few women will get breast

---

* Britain's "Million Women" Study was larger. It was not international, however, and did not compare drinkers with non-drinkers. It also found lower rates of breast cancer.

cancer anyway whether they drink or not – currently about 1 in 8 women. So to judge the impact of any extra risk, you have to include the basic underlying "absolute" risk. Without subjecting you to the utterly dull mathematics at this stage,* a 1 in 8 risk means that women have a 12.5% risk of getting breast cancer willy-nilly at some stage in their lives. Assuming drinking causes a 40% increase in "relative risk", what's the "absolute" extra risk of getting breast cancer? 2% to 3%.

So evidence from the world's biggest international alcohol/breast cancer study, when analysed mathematically, results in the conclusion that that, if a woman drinks, she has a few percent extra risk of getting breast cancer. Harvard Professor Walter Willet, one of the study authors and a leading expert in nutrition and disease patterns, likens the extra risk to eating too few vegetables: "Advice to increase vegetable intake and limit alcohol consumption would probably have a modest, at best, effect on breast cancer risk", he says. [49]

A subsequent Willet study on over 100,000 American nurses[50] found that a whole lifetime of drinking was associated with a 51% extra relative risk of breast cancer at daily intakes over 30 grams, 23% at intakes of over 20 grams, and a trivial extra risk at intakes below that. "We did find an increased risk at low levels of use, but the risk was quite small", say Willet and his colleagues.

So that's it in a nutshell. You now have a summary of all the bad news about alcohol and cancer – except for some other cancers which I've left till last, as they are not bad news, but very Good News.

---

* See Appendix One for how these figures are arrived at, and a much fuller discussion of the breast cancer statistics.

Cancer: the Good News

Really? Yes, the evidence suggests you may be less likely to get certain cancers if you drink. However, because the whole idea of alcohol as a cancer preventive sticks so firmly in the collective medical craw, there aren't a huge number of studies on the subject. Nevertheless, there's enough data to be pretty sure that drinking will save at least two bodily organs from cancer – indeed, they may even welcome being marinated in it.

First, **kidney cancer** – the eighth most common cancer, whose incidence has been steadily increasing year by year, and now accounts for 3% of all cancers. But alcohol is in no way to blame – in fact, quite the reverse.

In 2007, scientists at Harvard University and the Brigham & Young Hospital in Boston did a massive synthesis of all the existing research findings investigating the alcohol/kidney cancer link.[51]

Collectively, the data involved the medical records of over three-quarters of a million people. This is what they found:

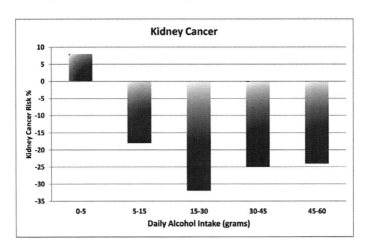

Derived from: Lee J et al. *J Natl Cancer Inst.* 2007 May 16;99(10): 801–10. Alcohol intake and renal cell cancer in a pooled analysis of 12 prospective studies

21

At very low alcohol intakes, the researchers found a very small increase in kidney cancer risk, but at higher intakes it went into reverse, with the risk decreasing pretty consistently with increasing alcohol intake – even up to a relatively high intake of 60 grams a day. But why? The 27 experts on the Harvard research team were puzzled. Could the nutrients in wine and beer have been responsible? No. The data showed that people who drank mainly spirits were also protected against kidney cancer – and spirits are just pure alcohol plus water. The logic was inescapable. "The finding that all three types of alcoholic beverages were associated with lower risk suggests that alcohol *per se* is most likely the responsible factor," the researchers had to conclude.

But surely there must be a point at which high intakes of alcohol damage the kidneys? Apparently not, according to a later Italian study on very heavy drinkers, which found the same results as the Harvard one.[52] "Risk of kidney cancer continued to decrease even above 100 grams/day of alcohol intake, with no apparent levelling in risk," they reported. So the evidence says your kidneys may welcome a goodly amount of alcohol.

Next, gastric *aka* **stomach cancer**. Although there's less of it about these days, it's still the world's second leading cause of cancer deaths. But it's very unlikely alcohol is responsible, according to an international survey of all the research data available up to 2012, which reported finding "definite evidence of a lack of association between moderate alcohol drinking and gastric cancer risk"[53] – a tortured way of saying that alcohol is not much of a problem with stomach cancer.[*]

Indeed, wine lovers could find their drinking habits might even protect them against the cancer, according to top Danish researchers.[54] They tracked nearly 30,000 people for over 30 years and found a clear "inverse association" between the amount of wine drunk and the risk of stomach cancer, with the heaviest wine drinkers reducing their risk

[*]   A very small extra risk was found above an intake of 50 grams a day, however.

down to a staggering one-sixth of non-drinkers' risk. "Linear trend test showed a significant association with a relative risk ratio of 0.60 per glass of wine drunk per day" added the researchers. In other words, every single glass of wine you drink a day reduces the risk of stomach cancer by 40%. There's no drug, vitamin pill or diet that can even approach this kind of benefit.

There were similar findings in a massive European-wide survey in 2011, where wine was again shown to reduce stomach cancer risk.[55] Beer didn't fare so well, however, with a slight increase in risk at the highest intakes

There's Good News for your thyroid gland, too.

Although **thyroid cancer** is relatively uncommon, its incidence is rising inexorably, particularly in women, afflicting two per thousand a year in the UK alone. Drinking could "significantly" bring this rate down, according to experts at the USA's prestigious National Cancer Institute. In a huge study on about half a million people conducted over a period of 7½ years, the results were unequivocal.[56] "Compared with non-drinking, consuming two or more drinks per day was associated with a significantly decreased risk of thyroid cancer," reported lead author, cancer epidemiologist Dr. Cari Meinhold. "The risk of thyroid cancer decreased with increasing alcohol consumption, by approximately 6 percent per 10 grams consumed daily."

A review article in 2012 added yet more cancers:

> Clinical and epidemiological studies indicate that it is mainly red wine which may protect against certain types of cancer ... including basal cell carcinoma, prostate, ... lung cancer, ... [and] non-Hodgkins lymphoma.[57]

We'll come back to why red wine is so beneficial in Chapter 12.

So ... alcohol and cancer is a confused picture, to put it mildly. As we've seen, while there's evidence that alcohol is associated with four cancers, there's arguably better quality evidence it's associated with a reduced risk of at least two cancers. And with most of the 200 or so other cancers, alcohol has no discernable connection whatever.

Although that last paragraph is scientifically uncontestable, this is almost certainly the first time you will have ever seen it in print. What you may have read until now might have convinced you that alcohol is a major cause of cancer. The data say it isn't.

One of the reasons that the alcohol/cancer link appears to be so weak is because alcohol is not itself carcinogenic – although you'd be forgiven for believing otherwise, given the medical propaganda.

The current medical explanation for the alcohol/cancer link is a compound called acetaldehyde. This is alcohol's main "metabolite", meaning it's what alcohol turns into in the body. In the liver, an enzyme called alcohol dehydrogenase oxidises alcohol into acetaldehyde, and it's this chemical that is supposed to cause cancer.

However, there are three major problems with this theory. First, acetaldehyde is widely found in nature, since it's produced by plants as part of their normal metabolism – occurring at relatively high levels in coffee, wheat and fruit, for example. In fact, it's considered so harmless that it's a permitted GRAS food additive – GRAS is the food industry's acronym for Generally Recognised As Safe.[58] Second, when alcohol turns into acetaldehyde in the body, it's only a fleeting intermediate stage: the final stage is acetic acid. What's acetic acid ? Common examples are lemon juice and vinegar – pretty harmless, and certainly not carcinogenic. Furthermore, the body doesn't hang around while it reprocesses acetaldehyde. "The rate of metabolism to acetic acid varies, but it is generally considered to be rapid," says a US Government report.[59] In fact, the length of time body tissues are actually exposed to acetaldehyde is pretty insignificant – the chemical's so-called 'half-life' is just a few minutes.

The final problem with the acetaldehyde theory is that

the evidence that it causes cancer comes mainly from experiments on laboratory animals – and even then only at high doses administered via the lungs. The vast majority of studies adding acetaldehyde to the animals' water supply have shown it to be harmless.[60] Only one study, using very high doses, produced cancer in rats, but none of the rat cancers corresponded to the ones claimed to be alcohol-related in humans.[61]

However, there is some recent evidence that at first sight appears to support the 'acetaldehyde is a carcinogen' theory – because the substance has been shown to damage DNA. In August 2012, in what was billed as "the first study to prove that alcohol is carcinogenic",[62] Professor Silvia Balbo of the University of Minnesota reported finding evidence that alcohol "damages DNA dramatically".[63] She arrived at this conclusion by giving vodka to human volunteers and testing their "oral cells". She found that the alcohol became metabolised into acetaldehyde in the mouth, and that the cells then developed what are called DNA adducts, "which are known major players in carcinogenesis", she said. 'It's acetaldehyde that latches onto DNA and interferes with DNA activity in a way linked to an increased risk of cancer." This could, of course, help explain alcohol's effects on the mouth, throat and gullet.

However, Balbo was quick to point out that this localised harm does not occur elsewhere in the body, because its innate 'alcohol dehydrogenase' enzymes offer "a highly effective natural repair mechanism for correcting the damage from DNA adducts" – except, she added, in people of Asian descent (see chapter 10).

Another study – billed as showing "for the first time how alcohol destroys DNA" – seems to lend support to the Bad News about alcohol and DNA.[64] In July 2011 Cambridge University researcher Dr Ketan Patel reported giving "a dose of alcohol equivalent to a single episode of binge drinking" to pregnant mice, and found that their foetuses "suffered catastrophic damage". However, what was less clear in the press story is that Patel had used mice genetically engineered specifically to destroy the two enzymes which are the body's natural defences against alcohol. So the relevance to real life is extremely tenuous – a limitation Patel later acknowledged. "We (humans) have two levels of protection against alcohol," he said. "First, as soon as you produce these aldehydes, there's an enzyme that degrades them and takes them away. However, if they still persist after that and attack DNA, then there's a set of DNA repair proteins which fix the damaged DNA and restore genetic integrity."[65]

So the DNA problem appears to be a red herring, because the body's natural defence mechanisms sort it out – apart from during the brief moments when alcohol's on its way down to the stomach.

Thus, the evidence as a whole suggests that neither alcohol nor its metabolites are in practice carcinogenic – certainly in Western populations. So there's probably no biological rationale for alcohol causing cancer.

The implications are profound. The logical conclusion is that the supposed alcohol/cancer connection could be merely a spurious association, and not a causal one at all. Remember the caveat of the breast cancer researchers: "if we assume causality"? Well, there appears to be scant convincing evidence that we can.*

And yet most medical authorities use the Big C as the Big Reason not to touch a drop. Remember the *ex cathedra* proclamation from the WCRF Report? "From the point of view of cancer prevention, the best level of alcohol consumption is zero."

How sensible is that advice, however? If you think about it, it's about as helpful as saying: "To avoid being killed on the roads, stay in bed." And anyway the statement is not true, as the evidence of the benefits of alcohol for kidney and thyroid cancer – and wine for many others – attests.

From the point of view of cancer prevention, the data

---

*   Although see Appendix One for a discussion of this issue in the case of breast cancer.

show that the best level of alcohol consumption is not zero, therefore.

Other Conditions

Besides cancer, what other health problems appear to be alcohol-related? At the start of this chapter, the NHS told us that alcohol causes **strokes.** Well, that's true. Alcohol does cause strokes, but it also prevents strokes. That's not as crazy as it sounds, because there are two major types of stroke: haemorrhagic and ischemic. Drinkers have been found to have an increased risk of the former type, but a decreased risk of the latter – at moderate intakes, certainly.[66] That apparent para-dox means it may be swings and roundabouts with alcohol and strokes.

The NHS also warned about **high blood pressure**. That's true too: alcohol has indeed been found to raise blood pressure, although only above a daily intake of about 40 grams, according to a study on over 80,000 Americans.[67] However, high blood pressure isn't a disease *per se* (despite what the drug companies would like us to believe), and it's only a minor risk factor for things like haemorrhagic strokes. In any case, experts admit that the evidence that alcohol raises blood pressure is "inconsistent".[68]

Another NHS target is **pancreatitis** (inflammation of the pancreas). This can indeed be a bit of a problem, but only if you drink substantial amounts – although the risk merely doubles at 60 gms a day, and triples at 100 gms.[69] However, pancreatitis is pretty rare, affecting less than 0.3% of us (mainly men), so it's not in itself a huge health risk.

One issue the NHS omitted is **drinking in pregnancy** and the problem of what's called Fetal Alcohol Syndrome (FAS). Perhaps surprisingly, however, the overall evidence for FAS appears to be pretty poor, according to experts at Oxford University's Perinatal Epidemiology Unit. Their 2007 review of the medical literature could find "no convincing evidence of adverse effects" – even among binge-drinking pregnant mums – " except possibly on neurodevelopmental outcomes."[70]

However, absence of evidence is not the same as evidence of absence, so the fact that there's little high quality science in this area doesn't really say much – apart from "don't know". Part of the problem is that this is a very complex field with massive 'confounders' of social class, educational level, concomitant drug abuse, malnutrition and genes.[71] On the other hand, there's solid evidence from animal experiments that high intakes of alcohol can damage the foetus, particularly in central nervous system development.[72] However, "moderate" drinking by human mothers seems to do no harm to their babies, according to a large Dutch study in 2010,[73] which defines "moderate" as up to about 12 grams of alcohol a day. Nevertheless, the overall advice to mums-to-be is 'better to be safe than sorry' ... and why not?

So let's recap on the alcohol-related diseases claimed by the NHS. Remember what they were?

>high blood pressure (hypertension)
>stroke
>*heart disease*
>pancreatitis
>liver disease
>liver cancer
>cancer of the mouth
>head and neck cancer
>breast cancer
>bowel cancer
>*dementia*
>*sexual problems, such as impotence or premature ejaculation*

Well, we've already covered most of them, and shown evidence which, even if it does not entirely contradict the NHS statement, suggests that it's somewhat guilty of exaggeration.

The three italicised items I've not covered yet, because they're discussed at length in later chapters. As and when you come to them, you may care to reflect on whether the official NHS claim that alcohol causes dementia, impotence and heart disease is responsible, accurate or evidence-based.

Having waded through this chapter, you'll be pleased to hear that this is the end of the Bad News about alcohol and health. Most of the rest of this book tells you only Good News about Booze. But I warn you: the list of alcohol's health benefits is far longer than its hazards, so you're in for yet more of a slog through deadly dense data. But stick with it. You'll be amazed by how guilt-free you may feel about drink by the end.

3

Heart Disease

My wife's late grandfather was a Scottish civil engineer. Born into a Presbyterian family in the 1890s, he helped construct the trenches in First World War France, and spent a lifetime as a senior engineer with a major UK construction company. An exceptionally hard-worker, he developed heart disease in his sixties. His GP was another Scot who had little truck with modern pharmaceutical medicine, and prescribed his patient what Scottish doctors had relied upon for centuries – whisky.

He faithfully followed doctor's orders to imbibe a couple of tots of scotch a day … and lived healthily for another 30 years.

The GP was no doubt influenced by patriotic support for a fine national drink, but he was also responding to the widespread clinical observation that whisky is good medicine. Today, the evidence of a doctor's own eyes is frequently derided as merely "anecdotal", but in the days before formal medical research, that "what works" philosophy was wholly justifiable – and arguably still is.

In truth, most medical discoveries start with "anecdotes" and end with clinical trials. The alcohol and heart disease link is no exception, as a medical review article by the USA's National Institute for Alcohol and Alcohol Abuse acknowledges:

> Since the early part of the 20th century, clinicians have noted that coronary heart disease appears to occur less commonly among people who consume alcohol than among abstainers. Over the last 30 years, formal scientific inquiry has confirmed this observation.[1]

One of the most striking "formal scientific enquiries" was begun by experts at Harvard University in the 1990s, as part of their prestigious Physicians' Health Study.[2]

Over a period of nearly 13 years, the Harvard researchers monitored 12,000 men with high blood pressure. All the men were doctors, and typically didn't practise what they preached, some drinking alcohol at intakes way over their own doctor-recommended guidelines.

So what happened? If you had swallowed the propaganda, you'd expect the heaviest drinkers to have most heart attacks, and the non-drinkers the fewest. But you couldn't be more wrong. It was the exact reverse. Here's a graph of the results, showing the frequency of heart attacks among drinkers with differing daily alcohol intakes, compared to heart attacks among non-drinkers.

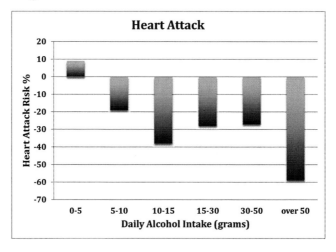

Derived from: Joline WJ et al 2007. Alcohol consumption and risk for coronary heart disease among men with hypertension *Ann Intern Med.* 2; 146 (1): 10–9

As you can see, apart from those who drank tiny amounts of alcohol who had a very small extra risk, the more these men drank the less their chance of a heart attack. Drinking 10 to 15 grams a day reduced risk by nearly 40%, and over 50 grams a day by nearly 60%.

Similar results were found in a 13-year Oxford University study of British doctors who also didn't practise what they preached, with a fair number drinking way above their profession's own guidelines.[3] "The consumption of alcohol appeared to reduce the risk of ischaemic heart disease, largely irrespective of amount", the high-powered Oxford researchers reported.

In fact, the evidence from over half a century's research seems to be overwhelming: alcohol is associated with a reduced risk of all forms of heart disease.[4]

This is an expert summary by heart specialist Professor Thomas Pearson of Rochester University, New York who makes the clinching point that post-mortems reveal that drinkers have considerably less atherosclerosis (furred-up arteries) than teetotallers.

> More than a dozen prospective studies have demonstrated a consistent, strong, dose-response relation between increasing alcohol consumption and decreasing incidence of CHD (*heart disease*). The data are similar in men and women in a number of different geographic and ethnic groups. Studies of coronary narrowings defined by cardiac catheterization or autopsy show a reduction in atherosclerosis in persons who consume moderate amounts of alcohol.[5]

Booze as Heart Medicine

Even more remarkably, alcohol can actually help people with existing heart disease problems; in other words, act just like a pharmaceutical medication. One survey of the evidence showed a staggering 25% benefit of alcohol in terms of death rates – quite as good as from the best drugs available.[6]

Indeed, a huge 9-year study conducted on nearly half a million Americans found that alcohol "significantly" prolonged the lives of people already suffering from heart disease, reporting that:

The largest reduction, in both absolute and relative terms, occurred in mortality from coronary heart disease among drinkers who, at enrolment, had reported heart disease, stroke, or some other indication of pre-existing risk of cardiovascular disease ... even for subjects reporting four or more drinks daily (*over 56 grams alcohol*).[7]

Embarrassed by such overwhelmingly positive evidence, doctors have been forced to explain why such a dangerous toxic substance like alcohol can be so beneficial to heart health.

Initially, many medics assumed that the positive evidence must be an artefact – i.e. nothing really to do with alcohol, but with other life-style factors such as diet, exercise or social class.

However, the sceptics had to eat their words when the results came in from a mass of "interventional" studies, where researchers gave alcohol to healthy volunteers and measured what happened in their bodies. By the end of the last century, 42 such studies had been done, testing "biomarkers" of heart health such as cholesterol levels.

The results were astonishing – again confirming that alcohol is as good, if not better, than many pharmaceutical medications. For example, the drug industry has spent millions looking for a substance that will raise levels of high-density lipoprotein cholesterol (HDL – the so-called 'good' cholesterol), as this is known to correlate with reduced heart disease. But the industry needn't have bothered, as regular drinkers had already got there.

A major review of the 42 studies showed unequivocal evidence that alcohol raises HDL to exceptionally healthy levels, finding that:

The average individual consuming 30 g of alcohol a day would expect an increase in HDL concentrations of 3.99 mg/dl compared with an individual who abstains – an 8.3% increase from pre-treatment values. ... After consumption of an average 40.9 g of alcohol a day for 4.1 weeks, HDL concentrations increased by an average of 5.1 mg/dl.[8]

So a comprehensive summary of the evidence shows that daily drinking at considerably above the officially recommended intakes significantly increases levels of 'good' cholesterol – a benefit unmatched by any heart disease medication.[9] There were three interesting details in the findings. a. Alcohol was found to raise HDL levels almost instantly – within an hour of ingestion; b. generally, the higher the alcohol intake, the higher the HDLs; and finally c. the least healthy people benefited most; in the studies, it was they who had the biggest increases in HDL levels.[10]

These findings alone would be enough to make alcohol a major remedy for heart disease, but since the turn of the century, medics have had to rethink their theories about heart disease, having realised that its cause is far more complex than simply levels of cholesterol. The new baddie in heart disease is inflammation, partly caused by low levels of 'markers' such as C-reactive protein, fibrinogen and albumin. So, how does alcohol cut the mustard with these?

Answer: very well indeed. For example, in 2004 Harvard University researchers tested the blood of nearly 6000 healthy drinkers over 65, and found that they had very low levels of the 'inflammatory markers' that cause heart disease.[11]*

All types of alcohol – beer, wine and spirits – were found to have the same beneficial effect. So it follows that alcohol itself must be the heart disease elixir, rather than any specific components of wine or beer. This seemed to be conclusively confirmed in a subsequent analysis of a couple of dozen studies.[12]

Interestingly, in contrast to current received medical opinion that one should abstain from alcohol for at least two days a week, the evidence suggests that it's regular daily drinking that confers the greatest protection against heart disease – "an intake of 30 grams of alcohol a day [has] an overall predicted 24.7% reduction in risk of coronary heart disease", said the Harvard researchers in 1999. This has

---

*   Although see Chapter 12 for more recent data from wine studies.

been fully endorsed by subsequent analyses of the data. An overview of the evidence shows that regular drinking at moderate intakes is associated with the greatest protection against heart disease, while irregular drinking (including, of course, binge-drinking) offers far less protection.[13]

Dramatic confirmation of that requirement has come from an in-depth study by New Zealand cardiologists on about 1000 people with existing heart disease.[14] The researchers found that a recent drink reduced the risk of a heart attack by about 30% – and the risk of actually dying from it by even more. Commenting on the results, US Professor of Public Health at Boston University, Dr Curtis Ellison says:

> These [New Zealand] results suggest that you should consume alcohol on a regular basis, perhaps daily. Unfortunately, most Americans do not have good drinking patterns, and tend to drink nothing all week, then drink heavily at weekends, which is a very unhealthy way to consume alcohol. The best pattern is regular wine consumption with meals every day.[15]

How does alcohol help in heart disease – even to the extent of preventing an imminent heart attack? The evidence says it works by preventing blood clots. This discovery was made in 2006 by another Boston research group who found that alcohol suppresses the most dangerous kind of blood clots – the ones which are formed when blood platelets are "activated" by injury to the blood vessels and become extra sticky.[16] Astonishingly, it's these very sticky platelets that alcohol has been found to be particularly good at neutralising. The Boston researchers found that the more people drank the less "activated" were their blood platelets – a straight line connection suggesting another direct beneficial effect of alcohol.

But the next question is this: how much alcohol do you need ? If you look back at the chart of the US physicians study on page 30, it would appear that any amount of alcohol is beneficial, with a virtually perfect correlation between alcohol intake and protection against heart disease. In other words, as far as your heart's concerned, the more alcohol the merrier, it seems.

However, since that study, many more heart disease/alcohol surveys have been done, and when they're all pulled together (in a so-called "meta-analysis"), the straight line connection can morph into what medical statisticians call a J-curve, because the graph of the data has that kind of shape.

A J-curve shape indicates both Good and Bad News: a decrease in disease risk at lower levels of intake, but an increase at higher. Here's what a summary of the alcohol/heart disease data showed in the year 2000.[17]

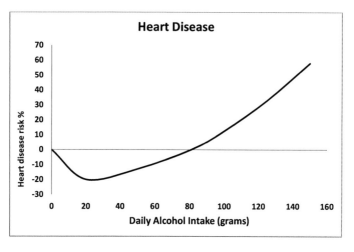

Adapted from: Corrao G et al. *Addiction*. 2000 Oct; 95(10): 1505–23. Alcohol and coronary heart disease: a meta-analysis.

The graph comes from a meta-analysis of about 50 alcohol/heart disease studies conducted up to the end of the last century. It demonstrates that if you drink between 18 to 30 grams of alcohol a day your risk of heart disease drops by about 20% compared to if you'd never touched a drop. It also shows that some kind of protective effect persists up to a fairly high intake: about 85 grams a day. Above this, the heart disease risk increases quite steeply – hence the J shape of the graph.

But it's fair to say many researchers haven't found this J-curve effect.

For example, one French study says that any amount of drinking is good for your heart.[18] It was conducted by two pukka scientists at INSERM, the French equivalent of the MRC in Britain or NIH in the USA. They studied over 43,000 people enrolled into the "2001–2002 National Epidemiologic Survey on Alcohol and Related Conditions"; fully 9,578 of these people were classified as "hazardous drinkers", and nearly 1500 were alcoholics. The researchers kept tabs on all the 43,000 men and women for a year, and this is how they summarised their findings:

> Our study shows that alcohol may have cardio-protective effects (i.e. *heart disease benefits)* not only in moderate drinkers, but also in individuals with patterns of use traditionally considered as hazardous.

Indeed, it was the hazardous drinkers who came off best, with an astonishing 40% reduced risk of heart disease.

Another study tracked 40,000 Spaniards for a whole decade.[19] It found even better news for heavy drinkers than the French study: "moderate" drinkers reduced their risk of heart disease by about 35%, but "very high consumers" had an even greater drop in risk, at 50%. Again, no J-curve, nor even a U-curve, but a straight line correlation.

Puzzling.

Even more puzzling is the fact that meta-analyses, which are meant to be the 'bees knees' in terms of incontrovertible health data,* don't consistently find a J-curve.

For example, the very first meta-analysis in 1993 by US researchers found that there was not a J, but an L-shaped shape in the data (there's a simple idealised graph opposite): i.e. that alcohol appears to prevent heart disease, but that heavy

---

* Meta-analyses are coming under increasing attack, however, for not being as objective as they claim/ought to be.

drinking neither increases nor decreases the benefit further.[20] So that's Good News for all drinkers, whatever their intake.

Eighteen years later, Canadian researchers revisited the whole evidence base – which by now had swelled to a staggering 4,235 separate studies.[21] Once again, alcohol's ability to reduce heart disease deaths was confirmed, with an overall 25–30% reduction. But what about heavy drinkers? "For coronary heart disease outcomes, *all levels* (my emphasis) of intake above 2.5 grams a day had similar degrees of risk reduction," the researchers reported. In other words, it was another L curve – i.e. drink as much as you like and you'll still reduce your risk of heart disease.

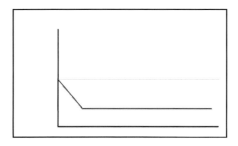

However, here's some less good and at first sight paradoxical news from that same Canadian meta-analysis. Although any amount of drinking may reduce heart disease, higher intakes don't reduce overall death rates, they found. As the report puts it:

> For all-cause mortality the association was J-shaped, with … an elevated risk in those consuming more than 60 grams a day.

We'll return to alcohol's effect on overall lifespan in Chapter 9. Nevertheless, the evidence is pretty clear that, if all you're worried about is not getting heart disease (perhaps because it runs in your family), alcohol appears to be the best preventive medicine around … and, of course, by far the most pleasurable to take.

4

Diabetes

Once fairly rare, diabetes is one of the fastest-growing health problems in the world – indeed it's now at "epidemic proportions".[1] It's hugely debilitating, causing major curtailments to sufferers' quality of life, as well as more severe problems such as blindness, heart attacks and even leg amputations. It's also expensive to treat, which is why pharmaceutical companies are now rubbing their hands with glee at the future profits lining up in India and China, according to a pharma market research agency:

> Factors triggering diabetes in Asian countries … are the rapid urbanization, drastic change in lifestyle of people … leading to obesity and naturally to an increasing diabetic population. The global market … is expected to attain a market size of $114.3 billion in 2016.[2]

$114 billion. Wouldn't it be nice if international health providers could save just some of that barely conceivable sum by reducing the diabetes in the population?

Well, they can … but how?

You've guessed it, of course: it's by prescribing alcohol.

There have been over 1500 studies on the diabetes/alcohol link, and, as with heart disease, it turns out that drinkers have a significantly lower risk of diabetes than teetotallers. That's not me telling you: it's the robust conclusion of a 2009 meta-analysis by researchers at Canada's Centre for Addiction and Mental Health.[3] Their review of over a decade of medical research shows unequivocal evidence that drinkers have a 13% reduced risk of getting diabetes.

That Canadian study followed an earlier Dutch meta-analysis of data on nearly 370,000 people whose health was tracked for 12 years.[4] This time the extra risk of diabetes amongst non-drinkers was found to be even higher – at 30%. So, as with heart disease, abstinence from alcohol seems to be a significant risk factor for diabetes.

Here's that Dutch study's graph of the reduction in diabetes risk plotted against alcohol intake.

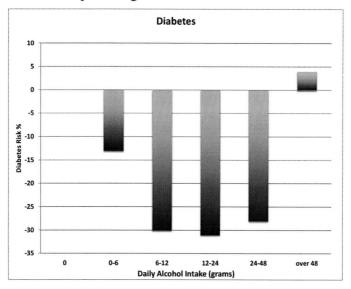

Derived from: Koppes LL et al. Moderate alcohol consumption lowers the risk of type 2 diabetes: a meta-analysis of prospective observational studies. *Diabetes Care* 2005 Mar; 28 (3): 719–25

The graph shows that if you drink between 6 and 48 grams of alcohol a day, you reduce your diabetes risk by about 30%. You've got to drink more than 48 grams of alcohol a day before your risk of diabetes goes back up to where it would have been if you'd never touched a drop. By the way, the Canadian meta-analysis thought that maximum cut-off figure was somewhat higher: 60 grams a day for men and 50 grams for women.

On the plus side for female drinkers, however, there is some evidence that, at more moderate intakes, they benefit from almost double the reduction in diabetes risk than men.[5]

And there's even better news from a more recent pan-European survey in 2012, which found that alcohol continues to reduce the risk of diabetes even at high intakes – up to 96 grams a day (but only for men).[6]

But another study says no: you're more likely to get diabetes if you're a heavy drinker, particularly if you "binge drink".[7] So there are some puzzling contradictions in the data about high intakes, an issue I'll return to later.

Nevertheless, the evidence is pretty clear that alcohol prevents diabetes, but how does it stack up against conventional medications?

There are two pharmaceutical drugs, Avandia and Actos, whose efficacy seems to be better than alcohol; on the other hand, they come with such life-threatening side-effects that few experts recommend them. Indeed, Avandia has been banned in Europe, and its manufacturers face an estimated $6 billion lawsuit in the US.[8] They are also very expensive. "It is impossible to justify [these drugs]," says Professor Victor Montori of the prestigious Mayo Clinic in a paper entitled *Waking up from the dream of preventing diabetes with drugs.* "If clinicians offer patients [these drugs] to prevent diabetes, they are offering certain inconvenience, cost and risk, for largely speculative benefit."[9]

Doctors can use an older drug called Metformin, but its long-term efficacy seems to be no better than alcohol, with a similar 30% reduction in risk.[10]

So, with so few drug weapons in their armoury, doctors' usual advice to potential diabetics is to recommend lifestyle changes such as diet and exercise, which tend to have a better outcome than drugs anyway. But if and when those fail, the research data suggest that the best medicine to prevent diabetes is alcohol.

So, how does alcohol work its magic with diabetes?

Glucose, Insulin etc.

As is well known, diabetes is an excess of glucose (mainly derived from carbohydrate foods) in the bloodstream, generally triggered when the body fails to respond to insulin, the hormone that regulates glucose levels.

What is less well known is that alcohol has some unique effects on this whole process. Summarising the evidence, a report in 1993 showed that alcohol causes the human body "significantly" to reduce its production of glucose.[11]

Although that's a short-term effect, it appears to have some beneficial long-term consequences.

For example, in 2002, French scientists did a comparison of insulin levels in regular drinkers and non-drinkers, and found insulin was almost 30% lower in drinkers.[12] Now, low insulin is a very healthy sign.* It means that the body is not having to over-produce it – either because there's not much glucose around, or (more importantly for diabetes prevention) because the body hasn't already got over-sensitised to insulin.

Alcohol was almost certainly the key factor in that French study because the researchers found that insulin decreased in step with alcohol intake. German investigators had come up with much the same findings a few years earlier, again confirming the causal connection. In fact, they found an astonishing straight-line effect of alcohol – even at huge intakes of over 100 grams a day.[13]

There's a graph of their findings on the next page.

Their data show that the more you drink, the lower your insulin levels. It's an almost perfect 'dose response', strongly indicating that alcohol is directly causing this healthy reduction in insulin. And the more the merrier, it seems, as pretty heavy drinkers have very low insulin levels – almost

---

* Low insulin isn't healthy for Type 1 diabetics, of course, as that's the cause of their problem. On the other hand, high insulin levels are usually a precursor of Type 2 (the far more common) diabetes. This is a complex area.

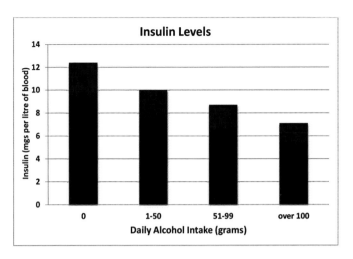

Derived from: Kiechl S et al. Insulin sensitivity and regular alcohol consumption: large prospective, cross-sectional population study (Bruneck Study). *BMJ*, 1996, 313, 1040–1044 (p =< 0.001)

half those of non-drinkers ... a staggering clinical benefit unmatched by any pharmaceutical drug.

But why are low insulin levels so important to health? It's because they significantly reduce the risk of what's called "insulin resistance". This is a condition where the body cells become insensitive to insulin, mainly as a reaction to being constantly flooded by the stuff (often because of a high carbohydrate diet). This forces the body to produce yet more insulin to compensate, in a vicious circle that usually ends in diabetes, i.e. an excess of glucose in the bloodstream, because insulin doesn't work any more.

The evidence strongly suggests that alcohol can prevent this happening.

But there's a puzzle, which keen-eyed readers may have noticed. The data about very high levels of alcohol reducing insulin levels doesn't quite tally with the meta-analyses showing diabetes is not prevented at such levels. Why?

No satisfactory answer, sorry.

This is just one among many examples of the inconsistencies in alcohol research. Having said that, however, I should point out that medicine in general is also full of them. That's because biology is intrinsically a somewhat inexact science (although Chapter 10 on Genetics discusses why alcohol may be part-icularly prone to such inconsistencies).

Meanwhile, back to the evidence.

Booze as Diabetes Therapy

Next question: what if you've already got diabetes? Can alcohol help? There's some evidence it might.

For example, in 2004 an international group of researchers tested people with already established 'insulin resistance' (i.e. a pre-diabetic condition) and found that 40 grams of alcohol a day reduced the resistance problem by over 20%.[14]

But what about people with full-blown diabetes? Sadly, very few research scientists have addressed this question. That's hardly surprising, however, given the advice about alcohol doled out to diabetics, who are generally told to avoid the demon drink, because getting tipsy could make them forget about their special diet.

However such nannying advice was ignored by Israeli medics in 2007 who gave alcohol to about 100 diabetics to see what would happen. The doctors played safe though, allowing their patients only a small glass of wine (125 cl) a day for three months ... but even that was enough to reduce their blood sugar levels by about 15%.[15]

Despite such promising results, however, no-one seems to have followed up on those Israeli findings.

So the totality of the alcohol/diabetes evidence is yet another Good News story to add to the heart disease findings. In fact, it's no coincidence that alcohol helps both conditions, as they are closely connected: diabetics have up to 4 times an extra risk of dying of heart disease, possibly because of their high blood glucose levels.[16]

And as we've seen, one of the first things alcohol does in the body is to stem the flow of glucose in the bloodstream.

This has yet more Good News implications which we'll cover in Chapter 7.

But before leaving the subject, let me draw attention to headlines that appeared in the world's press in early 2013, such as this one:

> "Binge drinking raises diabetes risk by damaging the brain."[17]

I raise it because it's a classic example of the uncritical, hyped-up news reporting on alcohol.

From the headline, you'd think that this was some new evidence about diabetics, revealing the shock horror fact that binge drinking caused their condition. Nothing of the sort. The story came from a press release about an experiment on mice by a bunch of New York medics at Mount Sinai Hospital. Their idea was to "test the effects of binge drinking", attempting to "simulate" it by feeding alcohol to laboratory mice for three days on the trot.[18]

They issued a press release reporting that the mice became insulin-resistant, and that this had huge implications for human drinkers:

> Previously it was unclear whether binge drinking was associated with an increased risk for diabetes, since a person who binge drinks may also tend to binge eat, or at least eat too much. Our data show for the first time that binge drinking induces insulin resistance directly.[19]

What the press release didn't say, however, was that, in order to create insulin resistance, the mice had to be given huge amounts of alcohol: 3 grams a day per kilo of weight. What's that in human terms? Well, the average US/European man weighs about 90 kilos, so 3 grams/kg translates into 270 grams of alcohol a day. That's a gigantic intake – particularly for three days on the trot.

But the science – and its reporting – gets worse.

In terms of the standard US measure of 14 grams of alcohol per 'drink', 270 grams equals 19 drinks. But here's the kicker. Binge drinking is officially defined by the US authorities as '5 drinks' a day. According to the scientists, the mice were made to "binge drink", having been given the human equivalent of 19 drinks a day. So how was the story reported?

"5 drinks a day raises risk of diabetes".

10 out of 10 for a sensational story, but the dunce's corner for science reporting. Another silly myth about alcohol was born, however.

There'll be more on the reporting of alcohol science stories in the last chapter.

5

The Body

1. Joints

By the time we kick the bucket, up to 3% of us will have got rheumatoid arthritis. RA is a painful inflammation of the joints, causing them sometimes permanently to swell up; it can cripple simple movements and make life pretty unbearable.

Although women are RA's main targets, it can also attack men. For example, at the tender age of 40, a brilliant electrical engineer friend of mine was struck down by the disease, forcing him into premature retirement. The poor man can now hardly move a muscle without pain, and his hands are gnarled and twisted into the kind of shapes you might find in a Hieronymus Bosch painting.

Rheumatoid arthritis is an auto-immune disease, meaning that the body attacks itself. Although there are drugs for it, they're not terribly successful, as it's essentially incurable. The disease is a medical mystery: no-one knows how or why it starts. "Currently, rheumatoid arthritis cannot be prevented", says Britain's official NHS website tersely.

But that's a porkie. Because, according to a wide variety of evidence sources, RA *can* be prevented … by alcohol.

Yes, astonishingly, the only known medication that can help ward off this crippling, death-hastening disease is the demon drink.

Have a look at the graph opposite.

These figures come from two separate Scandinavian research studies in 2009 which studied 3000 women, looking for a connection between their drinking habits and

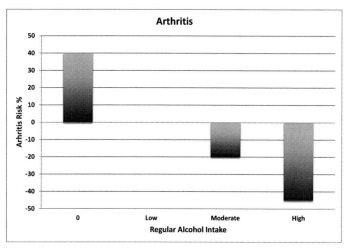

Derived from: Kallberg, H. Alcohol consumption is associated with decreased risk of rheumatoid arthritis; Results from two Scandinavian case-control studies *Ann Rheum Dis.* 2009 February; 68 (2): 222–7

their risk of RA.[1] It shows that, compared to the women who drank a little alcohol, non-drinkers had 40% more RA risk, but the heaviest drinkers had 45% less risk – i.e. a total of 85% less risk than teetotallers. It's a straight line correlation between the amount of booze drunk and RA reduction, strongly suggesting that alcohol itself is the direct cause of the benefit.

If this were the result of a pharmaceutical drug trial, the company would have long since been shouting "eureka" while popping the champagne corks – not least because of a hugely robust correlation at the level of "p = .0001" (statistical medspeak for incontrovertible).

But because alcohol cannot be patented, there's no way it could ever become a pharmaceutical drug for RA – let alone for anything else such as heart disease or diabetes.

Now, you could argue – as have some doubters – that these Scandinavian studies were only "snapshots" and not long-term follow-ups. To answer the sceptics, however, another Scandinavian study was begun in 2006.[2]

This one was very long-term, following 34,000 women for six years, monitoring their alcohol intake and development of RA symptoms. The results were clear-cut, showing that women who drank an average of 13 grams of alcohol a day had a 37% lower incidence of RA, compared to non-drinkers.

Pretty conclusive stuff.

Since those Scandinavian studies, more evidence has come along, showing that the most effective RA-preventing dose is about 10 grams a day. However, more is not better: drinking more than 30 grams of alcohol a day appears to be counter-productive, because RA risk increases at that intake.[3]

Booze as Arthritis Therapy

But if you've already got RA, can alcohol help? In 2010, Sheffield University doctors studied the drinking habits of over 800 RA patients, and again found huge benefits from alcohol.[4] The medics didn't measure the actual amount of alcohol drunk, but the frequency of consumption. They found that regular drinkers have significantly less severe symptoms than non-drinkers. For example, drinking for up to 10 days a month reduces pain by about 25%, and more frequent drinking by 30%.

Could this have been some kind of temporary anaesthetic effect caused by people getting woozy on the alcohol? No. There was objective clinical improvement, according to consultant rheumatologist Dr James Maxwell, one of the researchers. "X-rays showed there was less damage to joints, blood tests showed lower levels of inflammation, and there was less joint pain, swelling and disability,' he said.

How does alcohol work its magic on RA?

Once again, the humble laboratory mouse has been recruited to look for the answer, revealing that alcohol regulates "innate immune responsiveness"* to "prevent the development of erosive arthritis", say the Swedish

---

* For example, by decreased NF-kappaB activation, if you must know.

experimenters.[5]

Interestingly, both alcohol itself and acetaldehyde, its supposedly carcinogenic metabolite, seem to be equally good immune system regulators.

There's also some evidence that alcohol prevents RA because of its powerful anti-inflammatory effects. A pan-European study found people who drank up to 40 grams of alcohol a day had lower concentrations of C-Reactive Protein, fibrinogen, blood plasma viscosity and white blood cell count – all so-called "inflammatory markers".[6]

The evidence is crystal-clear, therefore, that alcohol can both help prevent RA and be of real benefit for people who have already developed it. But do doctors ever advise them to start drinking? No.

Neither do ostensibly independent, patient-friendly bodies such as arthritis charities.

For example, this is what the charity Arthritis Care tells its members:

> Alcohol may dull pain, but it's only a short-term thing …
> Alcohol also interferes with medications and can make any side effects worse. Steroids, Cox-2 inhibitors and non-steroidal anti-inflammatories (NSAIDs) have the same effect so, if you put them together, you get a double whammy.

So the message is that alcohol is dangerous because it "interferes with" drug therapies. That might be OK if the drug regimes were significantly better. But they're not. The fact is that even the most advanced modern drugs can barely match alcohol's efficacy.[7]

In any case, many RA drugs have serious side-effects.

Come on charities, whose side are you on?

2. Bones

Like joints, bones are another part of the body that degenerate with age. Osteoporosis, loss of bone mass and brittle bones are all familiar problems as we get older. But, once again, alcohol can come to the rescue to prevent us falling apart.

That sounds bizarre. After all, old people aren't very steady on their pins; that lack of balance plus weak bones is a combination that often results in fractures. So you'd think the last thing seniors should do is get tipsy.

Well, the evidence suggests that drinking can help strengthen old bones ... preferably while remaining seated, however!

There's remarkable data showing that alcohol can mend bones exceptionally quickly – within 24 hours. This was discovered in 2012 by US researchers at Oregon State University who studied a group of people very prone to bone loss: post-menopausal women.[8]

Their particular problem is caused by a lack of bone-protecting estrogen, resulting in excessive bone turnover. The women in the Oregon study were regular drinkers, consuming an average of 19 grams of alcohol a day, and they were brought into the laboratory to have their bone turnover measured by super-sophisticated X-ray technology. They were then forced to give up drinking for two weeks, at the end of which their bone turnover was measured again. It was found to have deteriorated markedly. They were then allowed to resume drinking ... with astonishing results: their bone turnover instantly improved, and within 24 hours reverted to its original low level.

Large-scale studies have confirmed these findings, showing that regular drinking significantly improves bone density in not just older women but men too.[9] How much alcohol is needed? The evidence shows that to obtain a 5% improvement in bone density, seniors should drink over "14 drinks a week", i.e. above 28 grams of alcohol a day. Is there a maximum dose? Apparently not. Some of the highest bone density measures are found in "problem drinkers".

What's a 5% improvement? It doesn't sound much, but it's roughly on a par with the most commonly prescribed anti-osteoporosis drugs … which of course not only come with side-effects, but are difficult to administer – they need a "very intense regimen", says the Osteoporosis Health Centre. However, as I've already suggested, it's not a good idea to self-medicate with alcohol if you're already a bit unsteady on your feet. Why? Because hip fractures are more frequent if you're a heavy drinker, for the commonsense reason that you're more likely to fall over.

3. Kidneys

We've already shown that alcohol prevents kidney cancer (Chapter 2), but it's also Good Medicine for the nasty little balls of calcite that sometimes form in kidneys, prosaically known as kidney stones. For example, a huge Harvard University survey found that alcohol in general reduces the risk of stones by over 20%, and wine about double that.[10]

Women's kidney stones have been found particularly to benefit from wine.[11]

4. Naughty Bits

> *Macduff*: "What … does drink especially provoke?"
> *Porter*: "Marry, … lechery, sir, it provokes, and unprovokes;
> it provokes the desire, but it takes away the performance;
> therefore, much drink may be said to be an equivocator
> with lechery: it makes him, and it mars him; it sets him on,
> and it takes him off; it persuades him, and disheartens him;
> makes him stand to, and not stand to…."[12]

Ever since the time of Shakespeare, chaps have been told that drink is a no-no for naughty nights … and the term Brewer's

Droop has been a firm part of the drinker's vocabulary for centuries.* But modern science says this may be – if you will permit the phrase in this context – largely bollocks.

The medical term for men's most intimate problem used to be impotence, but in order to sell Viagra, Pfizer's marketeers sensibly invented a less emotive term: Erectile Dysfunction (ED).

Since as long ago as 1976, researchers have been trying to obtain evidence to support the alcohol/droop theory, and had amassed about 20 studies by the turn of the century. However, collectively the studies have been a flop: while some do indeed uphold the droop hypothesis, most do not.[13]

Critics have tried to explain away this surprising counter-Shakespearean data by suggesting that the alcohol doses in the experiments must have been too low to produce the predicted effect.

So in 2006, in order to test this objection, researchers at the University of Washington did some necessarily intimate experiments on about 120 healthy 25 year-olds.[14]

This was serious science. Each man's vital organ was attached to a plethysmograph to measure changes in "penile circumference". Next, he was given enough vodka to get him drunk enough to be at, or slightly over, the drink-driving limit (UK and US), and then shown an appropriately arousing video.

What happened?

Permit me to quote the researchers at length:

> Contrary to ... conventional wisdom ... relatively high dosages of alcohol had limited impact on men's erectile responding.... An alcohol attenuation effect did emerge, but it was confined to one of five measures. Specifically, alcohol reduced peak circumference change, but it did not affect average circumference change, latency to change

---

* Brewer's Droop is a genuine phenomenon, but it has nothing to do with alcohol. It's caused by the hops in beer, which contain natural plant chemicals that mimic the female hormone, estrogen, which in turn counteracts the male hormone, testosterone.

onset, latency to peak change, or self-reported arousal. This circumscribed effect ... poses a challenge for the long-held view that acute heavy drinking diminishes erectile performance.

And in case you think the drink-drive limit is small beer in terms of intoxication, an Australian research team has tested much higher alcohol doses (at levels a notch or two below "producing loss of consciousness and severe motor impairment") and found no ED whatever – punching an even bigger hole in the droop hypothesis.[15] *

And I'm going to surprise you further. The latest scientific evidence says that not only is the droop theory mistaken, it could not be more mistaken.

It turns out that alcohol may actually improve sexual performance.

For example, in 2009 Dr Kew-Kim Chew, an epidemiologist at the University of West Australia, surveyed over 1500 Aussie males of all ages (from 20 to 80), most of whom were drinkers – of course! To his surprise, Chew found that the few men who didn't drink suffered from 30% *more* ED than the drinkers – even heavy ones:

> We found that, compared to those who have never touched alcohol, many people do benefit from some alcohol, including people who drink outside the guidelines. Even weekend and high-risk drinkers had lower rates of ED than those who drank less than one day a week or less.[16]

Of course, one swallow doesn't make a summer, so could this have been a fluke result?

Well, the answer has kindly been provided by a Taiwanese specialist in urology (i.e. the naughty bits), who rejoices in the wonderfully appropriate name of Dr Jiann Bang-Ping. In 2010, Dr Bang-Ping did a penetrating analysis of all the clinical

---

* Prurient readers may wonder how semi-comatose men could have been tested for ED. The researchers solved the problem by monitoring the men's spontaneous nocturnal erections, which were found to persist despite very high blood alcohol levels.

evidence for alcohol's effect on male virility, comprising about 20 separate studies conducted all over the world.[17]

Although research on three male populations (Koreans, Japanese and heavy-drinking Belgians) confirmed the celebrated Shakespearean epigram, the rest of the studies found no connection at all. In fact, many found that alcohol actually seems to prevent ED – just as in Dr Chew's Oz survey.

Summarising the international evidence, the data show that drinking up to about 40 grams of alcohol day can roughly *halve the risk* of ED.* In other words, to keep your end up, carry on drinking … but stop at about half a bottle of wine a day.

Now you could argue that this benefit might simply be due to the fact that alcohol reduces sexual inhibition; but the evidence says it does much more than that. Alcohol turns out to have actual physical effects on the target organ – in fact, very similar effects to Viagra. Both alcohol and Viagra increase the body's production of Nitric Oxide, the natural body chemical that is intimately involved in male erections.

How do we know this? Once again, courtesy of the rat-arsed laboratory rat who this time may finally have been rewarded with a bit of a romp.[18]

But of course the Bard is rarely wrong, and there are indeed some unfortunates for whom booze is indeed a downer … utterly predictably, these men are alcoholics. Once again, I am indebted to Dr Bang-Ping, who reveals that "many alcoholics suffer from ED even after years of sobriety, [sometimes] characterised by … testicular atrophy and gynecomastia (*enlarged breasts*)."

Shakespeare would have phrased it better no doubt, but men are duly warned about alcoholism: impotence is bad enough, but shrunken goolies and man boobs? No thanks. (See Chapter 11 on how to avoid becoming an alcoholic).

Talking of feminine matters, what about the fairer sex's relationship with booze in the bed department?

---

* However, there is some evidence that men's orgasms are delayed by drink – even at levels below the drink-drive limit.

It may surprise you to learn that the secrets of women's intimate responses to alcohol are considered to be as worthy of in-depth scientific investigation as men's. Such research has been going on since the 1970s, and the current world experts appear to be the Washington University scientists mentioned above.

In summary, their conclusions are that, for women, alcohol increases the desire, but anaesthetises the performance – where have we heard that before?

In order to spare both my and my female readers' blushes, I shall hand the explanation of these intimate findings over to the researchers themselves:

> It has become well established through controlled experimentation that acute alcohol intoxication heightens women's self-reported sexual arousal ... to erotic films depicting explicit scenes of heterosexual intercourse. ... The effect has been observed with varying dosages [of alcohol], although generally it is more evident with higher dosages ... Paradoxically, there is considerable evidence indicating that alcohol can have opposite – i.e. attenuating – effects on physiological indices of vaginal responding ... [using measures of] Vaginal Pulse Amplitude. Across eight studies, all but three revealed that alcohol reduced genital arousal, with the effect being more evident at higher dosages.[19]

For women therefore, Shakespeare's famous epigram appears to have been amply confirmed by modern science. But curiously not at all for men.

Is it too silly to suggest that either the Bard has been misinterpreted for centuries ... or perhaps that he was being politely unisex?

Yes.

5. Naughtyish Bits (Men only)

One of the other bits and pieces in this neck of the woods is the male gland called the Prostate. This is generally described as a walnut-sized organ which only gets called upon during sexual orgasm; so for 99.9% of a man's life it does damn all. It matters not if you believe in the concept of Intelligent Design, or its secular cousin Evolution, the fact is that both of them have done a crummy job with this particular organ. The problem is that, as the prostate ages, it often gets larger. The medical term is Benign Prostatic Hyperplasia (BPH), although the medic who called it benign needs his head examining; it's only benign in that it's not cancer, but it interferes with peeing, and *in extremis* completely blocks the urinary flow. Damn annoying, very painful, and potentially fatal.

As this is a very common condition in men over 50, the drug industry has developed a quiver-full of medications, most of which seem to work, but at the price of a range of side-effects – including the dreaded ED.

As ever, prevention is bound to be better than cure, therefore. The trouble is there aren't any medications … except for … again, you've guessed it: alcohol.

The first hint that drink might prevent this most troubling of male conditions came out of the blue in 1985 in Boston, USA. Doctors from Harvard and Massachusetts General Hospital had been tracking over 2000 oldish men for over decade, looking for any connections between their lifestyles and their health. Lo and behold, up came the intriguing observation that the drinkers among them got less BPH.[20]

Since then, about twenty studies have been done, involving a total of 120,000 men from all over the world. Result? No question of it: alcohol prevents BPH … not in every case, but enough to make alcohol a reasonably effective medication, reducing the risk of BPH by up to 35%. How much alcohol do you need to get that level of protection? "36 grams a day or greater", say US experts.[21]

So cheers, chaps ! Medical science tells us that saying "down the hatch" may really be of benefit ... down near our biologically most fundamental hatch!*

---

* However, BPH is not the same as prostate cancer, where there is contradictory evidence about alcohol's role – as ever, on the one hand, on the other. ....

6

The Brain

Every drinker knows too much booze does your head in. The lexicon says it all: addled, blotto, legless, paralytic, plastered, pole-axed, ruined, slaughtered, sloshed, sizzled, smashed, spaced-out, spifflicated, squiffy, tiddly, tipsy, trashed, trollied, wasted, wiped out, woozy, wrecked, zombied, zonked.

But this chapter could blow your mind even while you're stone cold sober ... because modern medical science says that what alcohol does to your brain can be seriously beneficial; yes, beneficial.

That's odd because alcohol is a powerful mind-altering drug, and potentially toxic too.

Of course, if you're an alcoholic on Skid Row or in the Savoy, it's possible your brain cells may long since be damaged, because scientific research says alcohol can cause "neurodegeneration through multiple mechanisms and in multiple brain regions."[1]

Adolescent binge-drinking is claimed to create similar neurological havoc ... or at least that's what happens in the brains of bingeing laboratory rats.[2]

Until the advent of brain scans, the only really solid evidence we had about human brains and alcohol damage came from autopsies, which merely showed that alcoholics' brains were slightly shrunken.

But MRI scanning has changed all that, revealing that some alcoholics have "white matter loss" in various parts of the brain such as the cortex, plus some damage to frontal lobes.[3]

Fortunately, however, the damage appears to be reversible: if alcoholics stop drinking, the brain seems to be able to repair itself – and quite fast too.[4]

In about 13% of alcoholics, some researchers have found visible evidence of a condition called Wernicke–Korsakoff Syndrome, which kills brain cells and damages white matter.[5] However WKS is mainly caused by a deficiency of vitamin B1, which is a well-known side-effect of alcoholism, so it's not the alcohol itself that appears to do the direct brain damage.

In truth, however, this is all a bit of a grey area, as fully half of alcoholics have no signs of cognitive problems whatever, let alone brain damage.[6] So alcohol appears not to be quite the universal destroyer of brain cells we might have imagined.

What's even more surprising is that normal drinking can actually help the brain by increasing brain cell production.

Really?

1. Brain Power

Once again, we have the laboratory rat to thank for this counter-intuitive Good News about the brain. In 2005, scientists at Sweden's famous Karolinska Institute came up with the astonishing finding that alcohol, if consumed at "moderate" levels over a relatively long time period, "enhances the formation of new cells in the adult brain".[7]

It's already well known that the brain is constantly renewing its own cells, but this evidence says that alcohol gives the whole process a useful fillip.

How much alcohol do you need to drink to obtain this welcome boost of brain cells? Well, the lab rats' consumption corresponded to "that found in normal social situations," say the Swedish scientists. So, the implication is: to keep yourself mentally firing on four cylinders, don't pass up those dinner/cocktail party invitations.

Interestingly, the Swedes found that the extra cell production was mainly in the area of the brain called the dentate gyrus, which is involved with memory and learning.

What's more, these beneficial changes were found to be "long-lasting", with a permanent increase in brain cell numbers, even days after alcohol was withdrawn from the rats.

So what though? Rats aren't humans. But tests with people show very much the same thing. Take some very interesting research on British civil servants (who, despite their public reputation, do classify as human!) done by researchers at London's prestigious University College (UCL) in the early part of this century.[8]

Research-wise, civil servants are a useful bunch, as they are the next best thing to laboratory rats: they're office-caged, they tend to be conformist and obedient, and often lead predictable lives; they also have an advantage in that their rigid job grade structure mean they can be studied across the social class/education strata.

The UCL researchers studied 6000 male and female Whitehall-based civil servants for over 11 years, noting their alcohol intake and testing their mental functioning. The first striking thing to emerge from their study is the massive differences in alcohol intake between the job groups, with the top grades drinking three times as much as the bottom ones. And, although most were moderate drinkers, a good 10% of the top grade males had intakes above their government masters' guidelines, at over 35 grams of alcohol a day.

There was a similar alcohol intake/job grade connection among female civil servants, although they drank much less than the men.

What about the human rodents' mental abilities though?

The civil servants were given five different tests of 'cognitive function': the two standard Verbal and Non-verbal IQ ones, plus three tests of memory and verbal fluency.

As expected, the highest grade people scored highest on all tests. No surprise there. But the truly astonishing finding was that alcohol intake was more strongly associated with mental functioning than job status. It was how much they drank, not their pay grade which most closely matched the test results.

Opposite is a graph of the mental functioning test data for the male civil servants, with *all job grades* pooled together. What's really striking is a clear improvement in mental functioning with increasing alcohol intake. Apart from a minor blip at an intake of 24–36 grams a day, it's an almost straight-line increase.

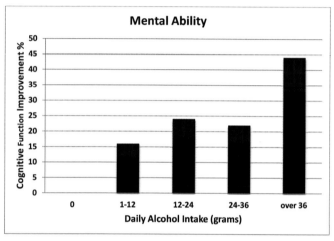

Derived from: Britton, A et al., Alcohol Consumption and Cognitive Function in the Whitehall II Study. *Am J Epidemiol.* 2004; 160: 240–247

Astonishing.

Even more astonishing is the data from teetotallers: the men who never touched a drop had the worst mental functioning of all (not shown). Their mental agility was roughly 50% below that of the lightest drinkers.

Now, on the face of it, you could argue that this study isn't worth the paper it's written on. Why? Because it's potentially shot through with holes – in particular, how can you separate the effect of alcohol from the obvious 'confounding' factors such as social class, genetic intelligence, income, diet and physical health?

Well, the UCL researchers weren't fools, so they took steps not to fall into that trap ... by making full allowances for the problem. In fact, the graph above is an analysis of the data after all these possible snafus had been taken into account. "After adjustment for the confounders", the researchers stated, "our results appear to suggest some specificity in the association between alcohol consumption and cognitive ability."

Or in plain language: booze can make you brighter.

How much alcohol, though?

Once again, as with all Good News evidence about alcohol, can you have too much of a Good Thing? Is there a limit to the amount you can drink before the extra mental shine wears off?

Let's look at the intakes of those high-functioning Whitehall civil servants. They weren't exactly heavy drinkers, with only a few exceeding the recommended daily maximum. So their performance, as measured by the UCL researchers, allows us therefore to be pretty sure that 35 grams of alcohol a day will vastly improve your mental functioning.

Vastly? Yes, that's no exaggeration. The researchers didn't publish the actual percentage improvements, preferring to show the data in the form of the likelihood of being in the lowest functioning group. But on this analysis, the UCL data shows you're roughly four times more likely to be intellectually high-functioning if you drink 35 grams of alcohol a day than if you don't.

That's a truly staggering difference, which it's hard to conceive of any educational or social intervention getting anywhere near matching.

But what about drinking more than that? Will the benefit increase proportionately ... or fall off a cliff?

Clearly, if you're so plastered that you're chucking up in the gutter, it's hardly an ideal time to apply for membership of Mensa. But what about when you've sobered up? Would all that booze have damaged your brain, or might your IQ have improved?

Surprisingly, there's precious little research data on the subject. Sussex University scientists appear to be some of the few researchers to have tested the mental abilities of really heavy drinkers.[9]

Actually, these were so-called "binge drinkers" – a term for which there's even a formal description: in the UK, you're officially "bingeing" if you're a woman who downs 56 grams of alcohol, or a man 70 grams … all inside two hours.

You'd have thought that level of intake would really clobber brain function – but utterly surprisingly, it doesn't. The Sussex researchers found no significant mental impairments, and on some tests, such as the 'visual search matching task', binge drinkers actually scored higher than non-drinkers.

Leaving binge-drinking to one side, what is the overall consensus about alcohol and mental functioning?

That's not an easy question to answer, mainly because the research data is so varied. However, US researchers at the University of Chicago have collated the results of all the studies published across the world on the whole issue of alcohol and cognition – 143 studies in all, involving a total of over 400,000 people.[10]

Despite being hampered by the wide variety of IQ-type tests used, as well as by the international confusion about the number of grams of alcohol in a standard 'drink', the Chicago meta-analysis of the whole mass of somewhat disparate data is fairly conclusive.

It shows that on average the maximum cognitive benefit from alcohol occurs at "moderate" drinking levels, classified as 2 to 3 US 'drinks' a day, which translates into between 28 and 42 grams – an intake which the data says improves cognition by about 30% compared to not drinking at all.

Above that intake, the benefit gradually tails off, however, reverting to teetotal levels of mental functioning at about 70 grams a day.

Next question: what type of alcohol is best at improving mental functioning? On the basis of the evidence, the Chicago researchers concluded that the most beneficial is wine.

2. Declining Brain Power

Because of these very positive findings, recent research has shifted away from trying to dish the dirt on alcohol's effects on the brain, and has done a dramatic U-turn. The question experts are now asking is: might alcohol help *protect* the brain?

The spur has been our increasing longevity, and the fact that the health of our brains often fails to keep up with that of our bodies. As a result, many old people today suffer from 'cognitive impairment' – ranging from the so-called 'mild' form to full-blown dementia such as Alzheimer's Disease.

On the face of it, investigating whether alcohol might prevent dementia is a bit like seeing if a nuclear weapon could prevent radiation sickness. After all, there's a theory that heavy drinking may actually cause dementia; indeed there's a supposed condition called ARD – alcohol-related dementia.[11]

And yet, from about the turn of this century, there has been an explosion of research exploring the possible benefits of alcohol for seniors.

For example, in the late 1990s, American scientists studied about 6000 women in care homes, all over age 65; some were drinkers, others not.[12] The women, who were all of sound mind at the start of the study, were tracked for over 6 years; their alcohol intake was noted, plus the date of the first diagnosis of dementia. The results couldn't have been clearer.

In terms of who got dementia first, in pole position were the teetotallers. The women who drank up 14 grams of alcohol a day obtained some protection, but those who drank more than that *halved their risk* of dementia compared to non-drinkers.

In case you might think those findings were a fluke, there was a similar study published the same year.[13] University of Pittsburgh academics followed about 1000 pensioners for an average of seven years, giving them IQ-type tests every so often. At the start of the study, none of them were in care homes, but by the end, some had developed dementia. Look at this graph showing how alcohol affected the onset of the disease:

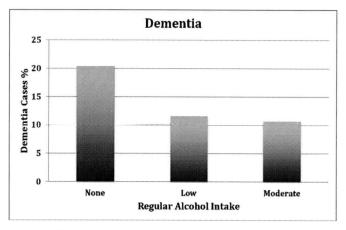

Derived from Ganguli M et al. Alcohol consumption and cognitive function in late life. *Neurology* 2005; 65: 1210–1217

At the end of 7 years, 20% of the dementia cases occurred among the non-drinking pensioners, but that risk was almost halved among the seniors who drank "moderate" quantities of alcohol – amounting to the odd glass per day.

A really startling discovery in this area has come from Germany where researchers did a three-year study of 3200 seniors over 75 years old, roughly half of whom were regular drinkers.[14] Once again, it was found that found that teetotallers had a much higher risk of dementia than drinkers. Even fairly heavy drinkers (downing over 40 grams of alcohol a day) benefited, managing to halve their risk of dementia. However, the most astounding benefit occurred with the old folk who drank a bit less than that – between 20 to 29 grams of alcohol a day. They reduced their chances of getting "overall dementia" by two-thirds, and Alzheimer's Disease itself to almost zero (a staggering Odds Ratio of .09 for the statisticians among you).

That said, not all studies are as clear-cut as these three, and there is some divergence between them (once again, biology is an inexact science). However, enough research has now been done (over 140 studies) to permit a useful pooling of the evidence via meta-analysis.

Since 2008, three separate research groups have done independent meta-analyses of the data, and come up with pretty similar verdicts.

That year, a British research group concluded that "low to moderate alcohol use in earlier adult life is associated with a 38% reduced risk of unspecified incident dementia," noting that wine at a range of intakes up to half a litre a day prevents Alzheimer's in particular.[15]

A year later, an Australian group's review of the evidence agreed, finding that "light to moderate drinkers" had a nearly 40% reduced risk of any form of dementia compared to teetotallers; heavier drinkers didn't seem to benefit, however, although they were at no greater risk than non-drinkers.[16] Finally, the 2011 Chicago review already mentioned concluded that alcohol reduces the risk of all forms of dementia by about 25%.[17]

Wine seems to be particularly good for dementia prevention. For example, a 2002 Danish study on over 1500 old people discovered that wine drinkers had about half the risk of dementia compared to non-drinkers.[18] A later French study went further, finding that drinking up to half a litre of wine a day reduced dementia by a staggering 80%.[19]

But, although the evidence is quite compelling, once again, there's the problem of causality. How can you be sure that it's really wine that's producing the beneficial effect? For example, the fact that wine intake is correlated with improved mental functioning could be simply down to social class: wine-drinkers tend to be both wealthier and more health-conscious than other drinkers.

However, we now have the answer ... for which, once again, we must thank the laboratory rat.

In 2013 Leeds University researchers working on rat brain

cells found that a major ingredient of red wine called resveratrol was able to prevent the formation of the beta-amyloid proteins that are believed to cause Alzheimer's Disease.[20]

But it's not just red wine. Alcohol itself has beneficial effects on dementia-related brain cells. The Chicago researchers referred to above were also psychologists, who often used rats in their research. They reported giving "moderate" amounts of alcohol to rats in their water supply for six days, and then looked at the animals' brain tissue under the microscope. They focused on the areas of the brain vulnerable to dementia, and tried to induce the classic beta-amyloid protein damage associated with dementia, using a tried and tested chemical technique. But they were staggered to find they couldn't induce the predicted brain damage. "We observed nearly complete neuroprotection," the researchers reported. "Alcohol effectively preconditions brain cells to withstand a variety of neurotoxic insults."[21]

So what does all this rat research prove? That there is a plausible causal connection between alcohol intake and a reduced risk of dementia.

This has been now been confirmed in studies of human beings. In 2004, Dutch neurologists used MRI scanners to examine the brains of over 1000 seniors, most of whom were regular, long-term drinkers – although at differing intakes.[22] None of them had developed actual dementia, but what the researchers were looking for were signs of incipient neurological disease.

What did they find? Interestingly, completely in line with the medical evidence, it was the drinkers who had the healthiest-looking brains. The data showed that widely differing intakes of alcohol (between 13 grams a week and 52 grams a day) resulted in maximum protection against "white matter lesions and infarcts", two classic precursors of dementia.

The really telling finding, however, was that teetotallers' brains had more lesions and infarcts than the drinkers' – again confirming the evidence that a major risk factor for dementia is never to drink alcohol.

But what about the heavier drinkers, the ones who drank over 52 grams a day? Unfortunately, the answer is not clear-cut, as there were two somewhat contradictory findings: on the minus side, heavy drinkers' brains had as many dementia precursors as the teetotallers', while on the plus side, two areas of their brains were found to be abnormally large – the hippocampus and the amygdala. Why should this be a plus? Well, the size of the hippocampus has been found to correlate with improved memory,[23] which of course is one of the first faculties to be lost in dementia. In fact, autopsies of Alzheimer's patients show clear evidence of brain shrinkage in these very regions; *ergo*, increasing their size is presumably a good thing. However, only 30% of heavy drinkers showed this benefit in the Dutch study, possibly due to a genetic difference.

In summary, therefore, there's substantial evidence that alcohol – especially wine – can help prevent dementia.

Booze as Dementia Therapy
Next obvious question: if you've already got dementia, might alcohol actually help to cure it? Unfortunately, no-one seems to have tried to find out – probably recoiling against the whole notion of drunken dements rampaging through care homes.

The nearest that researchers have dared explore alcohol's potential is with a pre-dementia condition called "mild cognitive impairment" (MCI).

In 2007 Italian geriatricians tracked about 1500 people aged 65-85 for over 3 years, monitoring their mental faculties. They found that, compared to non-drinkers, people with existing MCI who drank up to 15 grams of alcohol a day had a staggering 85% reduction in the risk of their condition progressing to dementia.[24] A year later, Chinese researchers found very much the same thing.[25] Incidentally, both studies agreed that daily intakes above 15 grams of alcohol were of no benefit.

So, the evidence says that if you want to arrest MCI, more is not better – on the other hand, none is not better either.

7

Losing Weight

This chapter heading is sure to surprise you. One fact that's been drummed into us about alcohol is that it's high in calories and therefore is fattening. It's a message harped on by the medical profession who, having scared us with their health propaganda, like to add the *coup de grâce* by appealing to our vanity. To fight the flab, they say, ditch the drink (my tag line, not theirs). The NHS Direct website asks rhetorically:

> Did you know a glass of wine can contain as many calories as a slice of cake, and a pint of lager has about the same calorie count as a small sausage roll?

Drinkaware says:

> Calories in alcohol are empty and extra-fattening

Here's a blast from the British Nutrition Foundation:

> Most people would baulk at consuming a full glass of single cream, but wouldn't think twice about a couple of pints [of beer]. But the calorie content is similar and, over time, excess alcohol intake is likely to lead to weight gain.

The trouble with these statements is that their message is just plain wrong. There is no evidence whatever to support the notion that alcohol itself puts on weight. Period.

That's hugely counter-intuitive, I know, because alcohol contains loads of calories – in fact, almost as much as fat – but the fact remains that alcohol isn't fattening.

I'll come back to why alcohol calories have no effect on weight later, but first let's look at the evidence in detail.

Professor Charles Lieber of Harvard University, who died

in 2009, is probably the greatest expert on alcohol and health the world has ever seen. In the 1970s, he founded the first scientific journal on alcohol, and was the first to establish a link between alcohol and liver disease in the teeth of a then sceptical medical profession. So he was no friend of alcohol. And yet he firmly rejected the notion that alcohol has any significant effect on weight.

As the first Editor of the hugely prestigious journal *Alcoholism: Clinical and Experimental Research*, Lieber more than anyone would have known his way round the medical data (some of which was his own), and by the 1990s, it was clear to him that if there's one thing alcohol is responsible for it's not obesity, despite what the calorie theory would predict. "Chronic consumption of substantial amounts of alcohol is not associated with the expected effect on body weight," he stated firmly in 1991.[1]

However, Lieber was relying mainly on inferences from clinical or survey studies looking for other effects than weight, and it wasn't until the 21st century that anyone actually checked whether the apparently irrefutable logic of: " alcohol is high in calories; calories put on weight; therefore alcohol puts on weight" is actually true.

One of the biggest studies was begun in the late 1990s, when US researchers embarked on a survey of almost 20,000 middle-aged women, whose drinking habits and weights were then tracked for almost 13 years. At the beginning of the study, all of the women started out as low to medium weights – (roughly, UK dress sizes 8s to 12s). However, by the end, the final measurements showed that about 9,000 women had put on significant amounts of weight, and some had become clinically obese.

Conventional medical theory would dictate that, other things being equal, the fatties would be most likely to be the ones who drank alcohol.

But they weren't – in fact, quite the reverse. The fatties were the women who didn't drink, and the skinnies were the heaviest drinkers.

I know you won't believe me, so – for the first and (almost) only time in this book – I'm going to run the risk of you falling asleep, and hit you with the full 'abstract' (i.e. summary) of the actual study.

Methods We conducted a prospective cohort study among 19 220 US women aged 38.9 years or older who were free of cardiovascular disease, cancer, and diabetes mellitus and had a baseline body mass index (BMI) within the normal range of 18.5 to less than 25. Alcoholic beverage consumption was reported on a baseline questionnaire. Body weight was self-reported on baseline and 8 annual follow-up questionnaires.

Results There was an inverse association between amount of alcohol consumed at baseline and weight gained during 12.9 years of follow-up. A total of 7942 (41.3%) initially normal-weight women became overweight or obese (BMI >25) and 732 (3.8%) became obese (BMI >30). After adjusting for age, baseline BMI, smoking status, non-alcohol energy intake, physical activity level, and other lifestyle and dietary factors, the relative risks of becoming overweight or obese across total alcohol intake of 0, more than 0 to less than 5, 5 to less than 15, 15 to less than 30, and 30 g/d or more were 1.00, 0.96, 0.86, 0.70, and 0.73, respectively (P for trend <.001). The corresponding relative risks of becoming obese were 1.00, 0.75, 0.43, 0.39, and 0.29 (P for trend <.001). The associations were similar by subgroups of age, smoking status, physical activity level, and baseline BMI.[2]

Let's unpack this daunting science-speak, and its even scarier-looking numbers.

For the purposes of this particular study, the women with zero alcohol intake (i.e. teetotallers) were classified as having a risk of 1 of becoming overweight – simply in order to establish a numerical base to compare complete abstinence with various levels of drinking. Now look at those 0.96, 0.86, 0.70, and 0.73 figures. These show that, as alcohol intake increased, the risk of becoming overweight went below 1, i.e *decreased* – and in a step-wise manner. The women who drank 5 grams of alcohol a day reduced their risk of being overweight by 0.96, i.e by 4%, 15 grams a day by 0.86 (14%), and over 30 grams a day by 0.73 (almost 30%).

And look at the even more striking figures on obesity. Here the study showed that an intake of 30 grams of alcohol a day and above gave the greatest protection, scoring 0.29, i.e. a more than 70% reduction in obesity risk compared to not drinking.

Remember, the 20,000 women in the study were all well into middle-age when the study started – normally a danger zone for weight gain.

So, here we have data that show that alcohol is not only non-fattening, it's actually in relative terms slimming. In the study, it was the women who *didn't* drink who turned into Size 18s, not the women who boozed. Drink *prevented* weight gain. Sorry if this all sounds rather repetitious, but the contrast between this utterly surprising but utterly clear-cut scientific evidence and official medical propaganda needs re-emphasising.

You're surely thinking "where's the mistake?" Well, if there is one, it's not at all obvious.

First, look at the consistency of the results. All the figures show a clear trend in favour of the proposition that alcohol intake prevents weight gain. There's an almost perfect linear connection: the more alcohol drunk, the less weight gain.

Second, the possibility that this was a chance result is effectively zero: those two separate (P for trend <.001) figures mean the results are to all intents and purposes incontrovertible. If this were a 13-year trial of a new slimming pill, the drug company would be laughing all the way to the bank with such overwhelmingly positive results.

Third, the researchers fully controlled for the obvious lifestyle differences that might have accounted for the results, such as exercise, food intake, and smoking habits. Looking at the data, they had to conclude that alcohol intake must have been the key factor – what scientists call "the independent variable".

Lastly, look at the pedigree of the researchers themselves: they came from the prestigious Harvard School of Public Health, and the women studied were in fact nurses. They were taking part in Harvard's unique, long-term study of 'health professionals'. So this was no tin-pot study.

However, this was just one piece of research. In the world of science, to stand a chance of anyone believing startling evidence like this, the results need to be independently replicated. That means other researchers have got to find pretty much the same thing.

Well, have they done so with alcohol and weight? Answer, yes ... and in spades.

Here are just a few studies conducted in the last 25 years which demonstrate that alcohol doesn't put on weight. I've put them in order of scientific incontrovertibility (adding the 'p numbers' for my medic readers):

1. "Alcohol drinking frequency in relation to subsequent changes in waist circumference".[3] [p= <.0001].

Who did it? Centre for Alcohol Research, University of Denmark.

How long? 5-6 year observational study

How big? 43,500 people

Measurements: Waistline and Alcohol intake

Key findings: Teetotallers and infrequent drinkers ended up with the biggest waistlines, whereas daily drinkers had the smallest. Drinking frequency exactly tallied with total alcohol intake.

2. "Alcohol intake and 8-year weight gain in women: a prospective study"[4] [p = .0001]

Who did it? University College Medical School, London

How long? 8 year observational study

How big? 49,300 women

Key findings: Women who drank below 30 gms a day were up to 24% less likely to put on weight than teetotallers.

3. "A prospective study of alcohol intake and change in body weight among US adults".[5] [p= .006]

Who did it? US National Center for Disease Control.

How long? 10 year observational study.

How big? 7,230 people.

Key findings: Drinkers gained less weight than non-drinkers. Women drinking less than 28gms of alcohol a day had half the risk of putting on weight than non-drinkers; men somewhat less. "Alcohol intake does not increase the risk of obesity", said the researchers.

At the risk of boring you, I'll stop here. There are at least a dozen other studies on alcohol and weight which by and large confirm the findings of the Harvard study on page 71. Not all of them show such a strong connection between alcohol intake and lack of weight increase (nothing in biology ever comes out 100%), but the general trend is in the weight-loss direction – particularly for women.

As a brief aside, I'll mention one study that bucked the trend. [6] It was done during one of those intensive medical check-ups often offered to senior management. These were 27,000 Korean men. Contrary to the findings in Europe, the men who were most overweight were the heaviest drinkers. Although it was only a snapshot finding, the researchers admitted they were puzzled, as they were aware their findings contradicted most of the European results. One of the reasons they suggested was that "Koreans and other East Asians have more sensitivity to alcohol than Western people, mainly due to genetic differences in alcohol-metabolizing enzymes".

That's a pretty cogent reason, because there are indeed major racial differences in alcohol processing, which we'll cover in Chapter 10.

Cause and Effect

But there's a major caveat about all this evidence: it doesn't conclusively show that alcohol doesn't put on weight. The data show only a *correlation* between alcohol and weight –

or rather, lack of weight. It doesn't actually prove a causal connection.

Although this type of correlation evidence is widely accepted as proof for the efficacy of medications such as vaccines, it won't wash if you're seeking to challenge long-held theories in science, whatever they may be. To repeat, nutritional theory is adamant that because alcohol is high in calories, drinking must *ipso facto* put on weight. To think otherwise is tantamount to heresy.

Fortunately, a few nutritionists have had the courage to question their profession's dogmas, and actually put them to the test.

In the last decade, a number of studies have been done, in which the alcohol and weight connection has been subjected to the kind of testing required to establish the efficacy of a new drug. Clinical trials have been done on healthy male (usually) volunteers who have agreed to be made to drink alcohol – poor chaps!

One of the simplest studies was done by sports scientists in the USA, who asked this commonsense question: does drinking a couple of glasses of wine a day put on weight or not?[7] A total of 14 men were studied for 12 weeks, during which they either drank a third of a bottle of '13% proof' (i.e. pretty strong) red wine a day for 6 weeks and then abstained for the next 6 weeks, or vice-versa. The results were as clear-cut as they were boringly revealing.

> In free-living subjects over a 6-week period, the addition of two glasses of red wine to the evening meal does not appear to influence any measured variable which may adversely affect body weight or promote the development of obesity,"

the researchers reported. So the extra calories from alcohol had no effect on the men's weight.

But that still wouldn't have convinced sceptical nutritionists. After all, the central tenet of the calorie theory is this: for weight to remain stable, calories in must equal calories out. So, the sceptics argued, if taking in extra calories from alcohol doesn't put on weight, it must mean that alcohol somehow makes people eat less, meaning that they simply substitute food calories for alcohol calories.

Although in most drinkers' experience alcohol tends to cause over-eating rather than the reverse, the objection had to be addressed. So in 1999, Swiss physiologists at the University of Lausanne tested 52 human 'subjects' to see if the sceptics were right. Predictably, they weren't: alcohol was found to "stimulate food intake" possibly due to "subjects [being] lightheaded after alcohol consumption, which might have had a disturbing effect on control of the size of the subsequent meal."[8] What a surprise.

Another theory the Lausanne scientists wanted to test is that alcohol might cause the body to heat up, and so dissipate most of its energy in heat (in medic-speak it's called "thermogenesis"). We're all familiar with the characteristic facial flushing after a few drinks, so a rise in body temperature could be a plausible explanation for the lack of weight gain.

So in 1992, the Swiss did a once-and-for-all study to test the thermogenesis theory.[9] Eight young male volunteers were subjected them to a battery of in-depth (and sometimes intimate) measurements while incarcerated in a laboratory setting. The researchers wanted to determine precisely how much energy alcohol actually delivers to the body, and how much of it is expended – in breathing, body heating, peeing etc – before it actually enters the body's systems. To make these measurements you need to subject someone to what's called "whole body calorimetry", where the energy of everything going in and out of the body is precisely quantified. It's the Rolls-Royce of nutritional research techniques – although it's not often undertaken because it's so expensive.

The eight men were individually locked up in a 'respiration chamber' for 2 days, and their meals carefully calorie-controlled. On the second day the researchers reduced the amount of food calories by 25%, but gave the men alcohol containing exactly the same number of calories, in order precisely to maintain the men's calorie intake. Would this "isocaloric" (iso=same) substitution of alcohol have any effect on the men's energy output?

If the researchers had been hoping for a breakthrough answer, they'd have been disappointed. Although they did find alcohol increased the men's body temperature, it was only by a relatively small amount, so the 'thermogenesis' theory couldn't begin to explain the lack of weight gain.

OK, they said, let's look at fat metabolism; could alcohol somehow be affecting that, and so prevent weight gain? Again the answer was no. In fact, if anything, the Lausanne results showed that alcohol should technically lead to weight gain rather than loss, as they found it "reduces lipid oxidation", i.e. doesn't burn fat.

The Swiss team was led by Dr Eric Jéquier, one of Switzerland's leading experts in obesity, who, at the end of nearly a decade's work, finally had to admit he was stumped:

> The relation between alcohol consumption and body weight remains an enigma for nutritionists. Epidemiologic evidence does not show a clear relation between daily alcohol energy intake and body weight. ... Alcohol drinkers tend to consume more energy than non-drinkers. Increased alcohol-induced energy intake with no clear correlation between alcohol intake and body weight [is a] paradox.[10]

Head-scratching all round, then.

So why on earth doesn't alcohol's huge amounts of "energy" (i.e. calories) not translate into weight gain? The academic journals are ablaze with competing explanations. The 'thermogenesis' theory was once the front-runner, but that's pretty well now been abandoned. Another theory: could the alcohol-detoxifying enzymes be responsible, or something called MEOS, the microsomal ethanol-oxidizing system? After sifting through the fine print of the data, those have been abandoned too.[11]

Another possible explanation has to do with insulin.

In Chapter 4 we looked at the evidence that drinkers have

a lower risk of diabetes, mainly because alcohol increases the body's natural production of insulin. But there could yet be more benefits, because insulin is potentially involved with weight control. How come?

Insulin's primary job is to regulate the amount of glucose entering the bloodstream; glucose is derived from food, in particular carbohydrates. Diabetics suffer from what's called insulin resistance, meaning that they cannot produce enough insulin to deal with excess glucose, so they suffer the effects of glucose toxicity. But in ordinary people, excess glucose doesn't become toxic; instead, it gets stored in the liver and muscles for later use. Crucially however, if those storage sites get filled up, the excess glucose gets stored as fat.

In theory therefore, because alcohol boosts the body's insulin production, the extra insulin should reduce glucose levels, thus preventing it being stored as fat.

Although that's a cogent explanation, the most convincing explanation for the alcohol/weight paradox has to do with the history of calories.

The Calorie Theory

Let me remind you what the problem is: alcohol is high in calories, which is one reason why we're officially discouraged to drink. However, the clinical evidence is clear that alcohol doesn't put on anything like the amount of weight which ingesting so many calories should theoretically produce.

To date, scientists have no real explanation for this apparent paradox. But this book is about to provide one.

First, let's take a look at a chart of what's actually in alcoholic drinks, in terms of the three major nutrients and calorie content. The figures below show what 100 grams of each liquid contains.

Calorie and Nutrient Contents of Drinks

100 grams	Calories	Fat	Carbohydrate	Protein

Red Wine	85	0	3gms	0
White wine (dry)	82	0	3 gms	0
White wine (sweet)	112	0	13 gms	0
Beer	43	0	4 gms	0
Spirits	231	0	0	0

The first thing that strikes anyone who's been watching their weight by cutting down on carbohydrates, is that the carbohydrate content of drinks is very low, despite their high calorie content. For example, red wine's 3 grams of carbs (at 4 calories per gram) is only "worth" 12 calories; but red wine supposedly "contains" 85 calories. Where do the extra 73 calories come from?

Even more strikingly, although spirits contain not a molecule of fat, carbohydrate or protein, they have a massive calorie score.

What's going on? Where do all these calories come from? To answer that, we must take a dive into history ... back into the late 19th century, when calories were first "invented".

The Clem

Of the many scientific terms describing energy, few of us know more than a handful: volts, amps, watts and calories. The three electrical ones are all named after real people, and by the same token we really ought to call the calorie the Clem, after a 19th century French scientist called Nicolas Clément-Desormes.

Clément wasn't a nutritionist but an engineer. His main interest was steam engines, and he wanted to find a more accurate measure of heat energy than horsepower. A patriotic Frog, he chose the system invented by his French countrymen – the metric system – and defined the energy needed required to raise the temperature of 1 kilogram of water by 1 degree centigrade as a Calorie. Latin: calor = heat.

However, Clément's physicist colleagues soon spotted a few flaws with his calorie idea (which I won't bore you with), and decided to abandon the concept in the 1880s ...

at precisely the time that an American agricultural chemist called Wilbur O. Atwater decided to take it up.

An ostensibly philanthropic guy, Atwater was worried by the poverty of the common people, most of whose income was spent on food. He wanted to determine which foods gave the most energy bangs per buck, so he could recommend the cheapest foodstuffs to shovel down the throats of America's labouring classes in order to fuel their toiling muscles.

Atwater wanted to sound scientific, so he stole Clément's "steam engine calorie" idea and turned it into a "food calorie" concept. To his way of thinking, the human body and its moving parts was indeed a kind of steam engine, with food as the coal and the stomach as the furnace.

To measure the energy within a food, Atwater decided to treat it just like coal, i.e. burn it to ash and measure how much heat it produced. And thus was born the so-called Bomb Calorimeter – a mini-furnace surrounded by a jacket of water, a device still in use today. To calibrate the heat produced, Atwater nicked Clément's formula: 1 kg of water raised by 1 degree = 1 calorie.[12]

Atwater tested a wide variety of foods in his calorimeter, and discovered that the three main food types followed a consistent pattern, with the most heat (i.e. in his terms, "calories") being produced by fats – more than double the heat output of carbohydrates and protein.

But Atwater was also a leading member of the anti-booze Temperance movement, the forerunner of the alcohol Prohibitionists in the 1930s, and he decided to see what dirt he could dish on alcohol via his Bomb Calorimeter.

The outcome was predictable. Anybody familiar with the stories of stranded (self-evidently wealthy) motorists filling their empty petrol tanks with whisky knows that alcohol is highly combustive. Indeed, alcohol made from distilling agricultural crop waste was a rival to petrol until the 1930s – and today's biofuels, of course, are also alcohol-based.

So, when Atwater put alcohol into his Bomb Calorimeter, it burned like a firecracker, giving off huge amounts of heat

– i.e. once again, in his self-invented terminology, loads of "calories".

Atwater may have hoped to derive some pro-Temperance propaganda from his Bomb Calorimeter tests, but they backfired. His results were seized on by the US alcohol industry which used them to promote the "energy-giving" properties of their products for the labouring classes!

But, of course, in the NewSpeak of today, high calories = bad, low calories = good. So alcohol is now firmly back in the dog house.

But calories are only a theory
We've become so accustomed to being told that such and such a food "contains" a certain number of calories, that we understandably come to think of calories as like little packets of energy somehow embedded within food. But calories are nothing of the sort. As we've seen, they are not real things at all: they are simply a measure of how much heat is given off when foods are burnt.

You may well ask: what relationship does burning food in a furnace have to what happens to food in the body? This was the question I asked myself when trying to work out why alcohol calories don't seem to count.

It turns out that not a single scientific study has ever been done to answer such an obvious question – for obvious reasons. It's just not feasible.

Digesting and assimilating food energy is a complex biological process which is impossible to replicate using laboratory equipment – particularly such a crude 19th century device as a bomb calorimeter.

Take another example: nuts.

Chock-full of fats and oils, nuts are among the top ten most calorific foods – in fact, they're often recommended to people who are dangerously underweight. However, in the last 20 years, study after study has consistently shown that nuts not only don't put on weight, they may even help reduce it. Nutritionists have tried to explain these findings by suggesting that nuts promote "satiety", i.e. they make you feel full, so you eat less food in general. However, at least two studies have shown this can't be the whole answer: when people are fed diets with identical numbers of calories (in the jargon, "isocaloric"), they put on less weight when the diets contain nuts.[13]

So we now have two examples of high calorie substances – nuts and alcohol – having no effect on weight. And there are other reasons to doubt the science behind the calorie theory.

For decades, the food/nutrition/diet industries triumvirate has rammed down our throats the message that fat is fattening and low-fat is slimming – hence the plethora of low-fat versions of virtually every processed food.

But it now turns out that the low-fat message is just plain wrong – in the jargon, it's "not evidence-based". This will surprise you, I know, as we are told that the advice which gets doled out by a plethora of official bodies like the NHS and the Food Standards Agency is based on sound science. And their mantra has been: "to lose weight, cut out fat and eat carbohydrates instead".

But the scientific and medical evidence says otherwise. I'll give you just one example of a clinical trial that proves the point.

In 2003, a US university team of nutritionists tested two low-calorie slimming diets head-to-head on a group of overweight women.[14] One was exactly the kind of type of weight loss diet recommended by the nutritional establishment and the food industry: very low-fat and relatively high carbohydrate. The other was the reverse – high in fat but low in carbohydrate. Both diets contained roughly the same number of calories, by the way. What do you think happened? According to conventional wisdom, the low-fat diet would be the obvious winner. But it wasn't – in fact, quite the reverse. The low-fat dieters lost 3.9 kgs, but the high-fat dieters lost more than twice that amount: 8.5 kgs. Particularly startling was that this group had got over half of their calorie intake from fatty foods.

Why are we so shocked by these findings? Because nutritionists have bombarded us with the idea that low-fat diets are essential to lose weight. It's a message that almost has the status of Absolute Truth. But I'm afraid it seems to be Absolute Nonsense – or more politely, it's not evidence-based. The study I quoted is just one among many which demonstrate that it's not fat that makes you fat, it's carbohydrates.

So where did the low-fat idea come from? Simple: from the entrenched belief that fat contains loads of calories. And who told us that? Our old friend, the self-taught American nutritionist Wilbur Atwater, with his crude 19th century food furnace.

To recap, when Atwater burnt foods in his "bomb calorimeter", he observed that fatty foods burned more fiercely than carbohydrate and protein foods, giving off twice as much heat – or, in his terminology, "calories". As anyone with a barbecue knows, fat burns very hot, easily catching fire. That's the reason Atwater derived the high figure of 9 "calories" per gram of fat – compared to 4 calories per gram of protein and carbohydrate.

So far so good – but so what? The heat measurement tells you nothing about what happens to food in the body. After all, burning a gram of coal creates almost ten times the amount of heat as burning a gram of fat, but no-one says coal "contains" 70 calories, and that therefore you'll put on masses of weight if you eat it.

The whole notion is absurd, but I regret to inform you it's an absurdity that lies at the very heart of the calorie theory.

The problem is that Atwater, whose basic theories, I repeat, still underpin modern nutritional science, made a fundamental error in thinking that because food burns, it therefore "contains energy", and that it's this energy which powers the human body. Nutritional science post-Atwater went on to claim that, if you ingest this energy (i.e. calories), but don't use it all up in powering the body's processes, the calories will be deposited as fat. Hence modern nutrition's mantra: to maintain a steady weight, calories "in" must balance calories "out".

You don't need a degree in logic to see that this reasoning is chock-full of empty presuppositions, one of which is: how do you know how much "energy" any particular substance delivers to the body?

Take the coal issue again. Coal burns far hotter than fat, and therefore "contains" way more calories. So why don't we put pulverised coal in cattle-feed to fatten them up? The reason isn't simply because it's unpalatable, it's that coal can't be digested by the body – in the jargon it's not "bioavailable".

Back to Booze

Now, you may think all this is a massive digression from alcohol, but it's not. To reiterate the "problem": alcohol contains loads of calories, but drinkers don't put on weight. Why?

If you've been following my argument, you'll have already got to the answer, and it's this: *the calories 'within' alcohol are probably not bioavailable* – just like the energy in coal isn't.

That's a line of reasoning only a very few experts can contemplate even raising as an issue, however.

> "The paradox of increased alcohol-induced energy intake with no clear correlation between alcohol intake and body weight has led to the curious concept that alcohol energy has a low biological value",

said Lausanne University's Dr Bernard Jéquier in 1999.[15]

The only other questioning voice is leading Swiss nutritionist Professor Paulo Suter who has asked: "How much do alcohol calories count?"[16]

But why do so few nutritionists raise the alcohol calorie issue?

Simply because the proposition that alcohol calories may be different from food calories is utter heresy. Nutritionists insist that "a calorie is a calorie", and proclaim this as unchallengeable dogma. As a result, the heresy is not only buried but ill-researched. By the way, this is quite common in science. Although scientists like to claim they're dispassionate truth-seekers, the reality is that ideas which contradict established views are often ignored – or worse, are so publicly vilified that scientists are too scared to investigate them.[17]

Fortunately, however, some scientists have had the *cojones* to examine the alcohol bioavailability question.

In 2004, nutritionists at Brazil's Fluminense Federal University reported on a series of highly controlled experiments feeding alcohol to young laboratory rats.[18]

In summary, they observed that the more alcohol the rats were given to drink, the less weight they put on – even though their total calorie intake remained the same. That last bit's really important. Obviously, if the rats had got so plastered that they forgot to eat, you'd expect them to lose weight. But the researchers measured each rat's calorie intake, and were able to show that each animal's combined 'alcohol plus food' calorie intake was the same as its 'food only' calorie intake.

There were five identical groups of rats, housed in identical conditions, and ingesting the same number of calories made up of food and alcohol. The only difference was the quantity of booze in their water bottles.

Look at the graph of the results on the next page.

These were young rats which were offered unlimited amounts of food, so they'd be expected to put on weight. However, when alcohol was added to their water bottles, their weight reduced in a perfect step-wise manner. Drinking a 5% alcohol/water mixture reduced their weight increase from 100% to 90% compared to the plain water rats, and this reduction trended almost exponentially. The rats drinking 10% alcohol basically stopped growing, and those whose water was laced with 40% alcohol ended up pale shadows of the plain water rats – almost three times skinnier.

And yet, I repeat, the rats' calorie intake remained constant, no matter what the strength of the alcohol/water mixture they imbibed. It follows therefore that the alcohol calories were not assimilated by the rats' bodies; in other words, alcohol calories are not bioavailable.

QED.

Although most nutritionists will find all this utterly unbelievable, it should come as no surprise to anyone who has read the evidence in this chapter and followed my arguments.

Let me quickly add, in the interests of science's perfectly proper requirements for 'replication', that the Brazilian nutritionists aren't the only researchers to have made such a challenging discovery. Remember the American mouse study mentioned in Chapter 2, which showed no link between alcohol and breast cancer? Well, the researchers also kept detailed weight records of the animals – and once again, they found that, when given alcohol, the mice lost weight, even though their calorie intake remained constant throughout.[19]

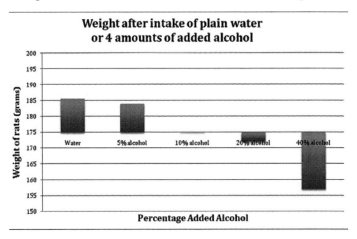

Derived from: Aguiar AS et al. Can calories from ethanol contribute to body weight preservation by malnourished rats? *J Med Biol Res,* June 2004, 37 (6): 841–46

A more recent study on mice in 2008 found very much the same thing. Nutritionists at the USA's prestigious University of Texas, Austin were concerned by the obesity epidemic among American women, and wondered if alcohol might be the culprit. So, to answer the question scientifically, they decided to test female mice, giving two groups either plain water or water containing 20% alcohol. To the researchers' surprise, although the alcohol-drinking mice consumed more 'calories' via the alcohol, the animals put on no extra weight at all. "In female mice ... chronic alcohol consumption did not increase susceptibility to gaining weight or becoming obese", the researchers reported.[20]

Now, you could be exceptionally sceptical and dismiss these studies on the grounds that rats and mice aren't people, and may have different metabolisms from ours. Well, it's certainly true that animal experiments have major limitations vis-à-vis humans, but these mainly concern pharmaceutical drugs, not foodstuffs. Also, there's the unassailable fact that most modern nutritional science is derived from experiments on animals. So, if you want to reject the alcohol and weight findings on laboratory animals, you'll have to throw out much of nutritional science's bathwater too.

But you won't even have to go there, because have a look at this:

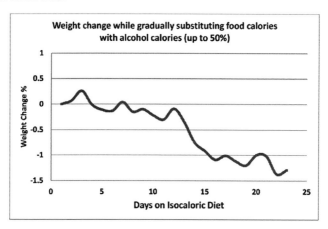

Derived from: Lieber C.S. (1991). Perspectives: do alcohol calories count? *American Journal of Clinical Nutrition, 54*(6), 976-82

This is a graph buried away in a recondite paper by the 'father' of alcohol research himself, the late Professor Charles Lieber.[21] It shows what happened to the average weight of 12 human "subjects" confined for over three weeks under "metabolic-ward conditions". For the first week, the subjects were given a standard hospital-type diet. On the seventh day, however, food items of a known calorific value were removed from the diet, and substituted by alcohol of exactly the same calorific value (i.e isocalorically). On each subsequent day, more food was removed and substituted by alcohol – again maintaining the subjects' identical calorie intake. The test ended after two weeks, by which time the calorie value of the food had been halved, so that the subjects were finally ingesting 50% of their total calories from alcohol.

In theory, the subjects' weight should have remained exactly the same throughout. But it didn't: the more that alcohol was substituted for food, the more weight they lost. As the graph shows, they ended up losing almost 1.5% of their weight – a staggering figure considering it occurred in just a few days.

Stunning.

According to the Calorie Theory, this graph is impossible – which doubtless explains why it's been kept from you.

You've also not seen it because the medical authorities probably didn't know about it either, and in any case want you to believe that alcohol puts on weight.

But now you know the facts.

————

That's the finish of this long but important chapter. At each bookend, I've shown incontrovertible evidence from human and animal studies that alcohol, despite "containing" many calories, doesn't put on weight – with the meat in the sandwich explaining why.

But I may be about to put the kybosh on it all … with beer.

8

Beer Belly

If you've got through the last chapter, I bet there'll be one big question lurking at the back of your mind. OK, you'll say, that scientific evidence about alcohol and weight may be all very well, but it contradicts the evidence of one's own eyes. What about the hordes of beer drinkers who may be able to prop up a bar, but are barely able to prop up their own bloated abdomens?

The spectacle of the rubicond, rotund, beer-swilling male of the species is a familiar one in literature. Dickens had Mr Pickwick, Shakespeare had Falstaff and Sir Toby Belch. The famous Toby Jug, depicting a bloated 18th century beer-swiller, is thought to derive from Henry Elwes, aka Toby Fillpot who suffered an early death, having downed 2000 gallons of a particularly strong ale called Stingo.

The beer belly isn't just a British phenomenon. The Germans have exactly the same word for it (*bierbauch*), while the French, with typical Gallic Germanophobia, call it *un abdo kronenbourg.*

So, heavy drinking seems to have some connection with heavy bellies – at least in the popular imagination. Now, I'm not one to dismiss commonsense observations as merely "anecdotal evidence", so let's address the issue square on. Assuming "beer bellies" exist, if what I've told you in the last chapter about alcohol having no effect on weight is true, what's the explanation?

Let's have another look at the beer section of that calorie/ nutrient table:

100 grams	Calories	Fat	Carbohydrate	Protein
Beer	43	0	4 gms	0

We've already established that alcohol calories don't count, so what are we left with? Out of the 43 calories "in" 100 ml of beer, 12 calories come from carbohydrates. Converting to measures we can all understand, that's about 50 calories per pint. Now, anyone familiar with conventional slimming diets will know that 50 calories aren't an awful lot. Even if you're downing the average pub session's 5 pints of "squeezy" (my wife's ugly name for the foaming brown liquid), you'll only ingest 250 calories from the carbohydrate content – the same as a single Mars Bar. Not much then, and certainly not enough to turn your belly into a balloon.

Clearly the calories in beer's carbohydrates can't be responsible. What else could be?

This is where I must introduce you to one of the most interesting nutritionists on the planet – an Englishman called David Jenkins. He's a Professor at Toronto University, and his mild English gent personality may explain why you've never heard of him. But he has revolutionised our understanding of nutrition.

Jenkins' area of expertise is diabetes, the condition whose sufferers have a problem with processing the glucose that comes from eating carbohydrates. In the 1980s, Jenkins decided to draw up a league table of carbohydrate foods, in order to show diabetics which ones were low glucose (i.e. ok-ish) and which were high glucose (i.e. real no-nos).

It was a massive undertaking. Jenkins realised laboratory tests wouldn't be good enough, and that only real people could provide the answer. So he got hold of a bunch of healthy non-diabetic human guinea-pigs and fed them hundreds of individual carbohydrate foods … one by one … in separate testing sessions. It was a laborious business. Each human animal had to have a baseline test of blood glucose, then be fed the food, and then have his blood measured every few hours afterwards.

After years of work, Jenkins' league table was ready. Each major carbohydrate food was assessed in terms of how much glucose it created. Jenkins used a numerical value he called the Glycemic Index (GI).

To calibrate the Index, he gave glucose a value of 100. All other foods were compared in relation to it. Thus, for example, cornflakes, being high in refined carbohydrates, scored 85, while less refined brown rice and wholemeal bread scored 50.

FOOD or DRINK	GI
Glucose	100
Potato crisps	95
Corn Flakes	85
White bread	85
Cereals	70
Corn on the cob	70
Banana	65
White Rice	60
White Pasta	55
Wholemeal Bread	50
Brown Rice	50
Peas	40
Grapes	40
Apple juice	40
Raw Carrots	35
Figs	35
French beans	30
Dark chocolate	22
Plums	22
Peanuts	20
Walnuts	15
Almonds	15
Green vegetables	10

So what's all this got to do with weight and alcohol?

Well, have a look at the bottom items in Jenkins' GI list. What do you see? Nuts. Doesn't that ring a bell? In the last chapter, we showed how nuts, despite being laden with calories, have no effect on weight.

The Glycemic Index is the only system to explain why.

Nuts score low on the index because when Jenkins tested

them on his volunteers, he found they produced almost zero glucose in the bloodstream. But what's that got to do with weight?

In the 1980s, a French scientist called Michel Montignac put two and two together. He realised that, if nuts score low on the GI list, and nuts don't put on weight, there could be a connection.

Montignac went on to write the first best-seller on the GI Diet[1] in which he cogently argued that, because fat is deposited in the body as a result of excess glucose in the diet, the way to lose weight is to choose foods which have a low GI, i.e. produce least glucose.

Initially nutritionists scoffed at Montignac's theories, mainly because he largely ignored calories. However, numerous studies have confirmed Montignac was right. It's now well established that low GI diets are far superior to conventional low-calorie diets, even if they "contain" the same number of calories.[2]

But what has this to do with beer bellies?

Well, I deliberately omitted alcohol from the GI list on page 91, so as not to give the game away. However, the bad news for beer drinkers is that their favourite swig scores very highly indeed on the GI chart. Montignac put it at a figure of 110 – yes, higher than glucose itself. Here's that (truncated) GI list again opposite. See how beer compares to wine and spirits, which are … way … way … down at the bottom of the list.

To be honest, there's been a lot of controversy about beer within the GI community. That's because Montignac's figure didn't come from actual tests on human beings, but was an educated guess based on beer's ingredients, one of which is maltose.

Naturally, the brewing industry has been keen to pooh-pooh beer's high GI figure, arguing that maltose is in very low concentrations in beer.

However, a group of Finnish researchers weren't so sure. In 2011 they brought ten volunteers into a laboratory bristling with blood glucose testing equipment. The result? They found beer's GI wasn't 110... but even higher: a staggering 119.[3]

FOOD or DRINK	GI
Beer	**110-119**
Glucose	100
Potato crisps	95
[...]	
Almonds	15
Green vegetables	10
Wine	**0**
Spirits	**0**

So here we have strong evidence from a controlled clinical test that beer does indeed have an exceptionally high GI rating, and thus is liable to be exceptionally fattening.

In principle, therefore, we have a cogent explanation for the beer belly phenomenon. On the other hand, do we actually need one? Where's the evidence that beer causes a beer belly anyway?

In the last chapter, I referred to a Danish study exploring drinking and weight gain.[4]

It was a massive study, in which over 40,000 people's drinking habits and waist measurements were tracked for 5 years. During that time, the men on average gained an extra inch [2.5 cms] around the waist, and the women about 2 ½ inches [6.7 cms]. But how much of that was down to booze? The answer was totally counter-intuitive. The researchers found that the people whose waists expanded the most were those who drank the least, and vice versa. Yes, it was the teetotallers, not the drinkers, who had to loosen their belts the most.

There were some interesting sex differences too: over the five-year period, the male drinkers' waistlines tended to remained stable, but the female drinkers actually reduced theirs. Indeed, the sveltest ladies were people our medical masters would classify as dangerously heavy drinkers, consuming up to 42 gms of alcohol every day of the week.

Fortunately, the Danish study was so huge that it could obtain separate belly size measures for wine, beer and spirit drinkers. Astonishingly, the figures showed no significant differences between wine and beer – not even the most serious beer drinkers ended up with a beer belly.

So is that the end of the beer belly issue? I wish I could give you a clear answer. Again, the unfortunate fact is that scientific studies aren't as definitive as scientists often like to make out – particularly in biology. Indeed, there's an awful lot of disagreement between one study and another about beer bellies.

For example, the results of that Danish study are flatly contradicted by another one – from Denmark itself. This time round, Danish researchers found that, although wine was innocent, men who spent a decade drinking more than 21 beers a week increased by 63% their risk of ending up with a waist measurement above 102 cms (40 inches), and for a woman a 153% extra risk of her waist exceeding 88 cms (36.5 inches). The researchers concluded:

> Moderate-to-high consumption of … beer and spirits was associated with later high waist circumference, whereas moderate-to-high wine consumption may have the opposite effect.[5]

In the USA too, researchers have also found evidence of a beer belly. In one survey of over 2000 people, the largest abdomens were found on heavy binge-type beer drinkers. Interestingly, they too found that drinkers of both wine and "small amounts of alcohol on a regular basis" had smaller waistlines – smaller even than teetotallers'.[6]

A similar survey of over 2000 Czech drinkers also found evidence of a beer belly, but only among non-smokers.[7]

On the other hand, beer drinkers showed no girth increase at all in a French study on 2500 people. By the way, the study also showed that those who drank up to a bottle of wine a day had a lower Body Mass Index and 'waist to hip ratio' than non-drinkers.[8]

However, a German study on about 20,000 people found that men who drank more than a litre of beer a day had only a modest (17%) increase in risk of having a larger "waist circumference".[9]

And a larger study by the same researchers confirmed that beer is the main culprit in "abdominal adiposity".[10]

This was further supported by a later Spanish study which monitored nearly 10,000 people for six years and found an increase in weight among beer and spirit drinkers. But it was tiny: a mere 120 grams (1/4 lb) a year.[11]

However, an earlier French survey of over 3000 people found that overall weight wasn't affected by drink – although an increased "waist to hip ratio" certainly was … on all types of booze, including wine.[12]

This medical tit for tat is getting really boring, so I'll stop.

There are scores of studies on the beer belly issue, most exhibiting the disagreements common in surveys, even scientific ones. When pulled together, however, the general trend of the data shows that beer does appear to have some effect on waist size.

Not wine, though. The data are pretty clear that there's no such thing as a wine belly.

But what about spirits? Keen-eyed readers will have noticed that some studies point the finger at spirits as well as beer. That appears to be a problem for the heretical theory that "alcohol calories" are phoney. After all, spirits contain nothing but alcohol, so how can they put on weight?

The answer is simple. It's not the alcohol itself; it's what alcohol does to your appetite.

Study after study has shown that alcohol is a powerful appetite stimulant. There's been some quite detailed research on this – a fair amount in Britain. At Liverpool University, for example, psychologists tested "12 males" in laboratory conditions, monitoring their food intake after drinking two different quantities of alcohol. On different mornings, before lunch, the males (almost certainly grateful students!) were given a canful of alcohol-free lager "spiked" with either 8 grams or 32 grams of pure alcohol. i.e. 1 or 4 standard pub measures of vodka.[13]

The researchers observed that the lads, who were allowed to eat as much lunch as they liked, tucked into almost 20% more food after drinking 4 measures than after 1 measure of spirits. Curiously, this effect persisted beyond lunch into their dinner intake – despite not having been given any extra alcohol to drink. They particularly went for tasty foods: ones higher in fat and salt.

A similar study at Sussex University found very much the same thing, noting that the cause of over-eating isn't the "disinhibition" caused by alcohol, but that alcohol seems to delay the feeling of fullness after a meal.[14]

Why does alcohol increase appetite? Nobody really knows. Unlike the hunger caused by cannabis (famously dubbed "the munchies"), which has been connected to a brain chemical, scientists have found nothing equivalent with alcohol. A relatively unknown stomach hormone called ghrelin is the current favoured candidate, but the evidence isn't at all consistent.[15]

Whatever the reason for the alcohol munchies, the research data offer a cogent explanation why spirits, despite containing nothing other than phoney alcohol calories, may put on weight and result in a "spirit belly".

But why isn't there a wine belly?

No idea, as nobody's yet done the detailed research. However, a study by psychologists at Glasgow University does provide clues. They found that, although wine increases appetite and leads to extra food intake, the body tends to compensate by reducing food energy intake over the following days, thus rebalancing overall energy inputs.[16]

But there's a problem: if there is such a thing as a beer and spirit belly, doesn't that contradict the evidence of the last chapter that alcohol doesn't put on weight? Not at all. First, beer bellies can be explained by the GI theory, so that's not an issue. Second, waist circumference and weight are two separate measures, and although they are frequently correlated, there's no reason in principle why someone couldn't have a spirit belly on a skinny body.

And third, as we've seen, it's not alcohol itself that puts on weight, but the extra food intake caused by the munchies.

Surprisingly, given the official propaganda about alcohol and calories, a 2012 NHS report on alcohol and weight agrees that "there is no clear causal relationship between alcohol consumption and obesity", going on to acknowledge that the real problem is that "heavy drinking leads to overeating [and] sedentary behaviour".[17]

In other words, too much booze makes you guzzle and loll. My point exactly. But it's got damn all to do with alcohol 'calories'.

9

Living Longer

You've got this far, so you'll now know that drinking can have major benefits for your health. To recap, alcohol will reduce the risk of heart disease, some cancers, arthritis, dementia, obesity and diabetes, plus a few more nasties besides.

So it won't come as a huge surprise to discover that the evidence says alcohol will help you live longer.

Of course, the medical profession hates to have to acknowledge this, as it undermines their negative propaganda. What do they do? First, they keep very quiet about the fact that non-drinkers tend to die younger, and second, they put up a massive smokescreen called "Alcohol-related deaths". Here's an example from a 2011 medical review:

> Alcohol has been identified as a leading risk factor for death and disability globally, accounting for 3.8% of death and 4.6% of disability adjusted life years (DALYs) lost in 2004. Alcohol was found to be the 8th highest risk factor for death in 2004.[1]

Another example from a UK Government document called *Alcohol-related deaths in the United Kingdom, 2011:*

> The number of alcohol-related deaths in has consistently increased since the early 1990s, rising from the lowest figure of 4,023 (6.7 per 100,000) in 1992 to the highest of 9,031 (13.6 per 100,000) in 2008. ... Alcoholic Liver Disease is the most prevalent of all alcohol-related causes of death and is responsible for approximately 66% of all alcohol-related deaths in 2011.[2]

Later in this chapter I'll show you the detailed evidence behind the statement "drinkers live longer", but for the moment please bear with me while I clear the fog surrounding "alcohol-related" diseases.

In the last few years, quite a few medical conditions have been classified as "alcohol-related" – from "alcoholic cardiomyopathy" to "alcoholic liver disease". This re-classification of diseases comes in very handy if you want to make a case for alcohol being dangerous, as it all sounds very scientific. Take this statement by a large international team of medical experts:

> These [alcohol-related] conditions are by definition wholly attributable to alcohol with an alcohol-attributable fraction (AAF) of 100%, where AAF denotes the proportion of a certain disease category which would not have occurred had there been no alcohol consumption.[3]

Or in plain language: the conditions we say are caused by alcohol are 100% caused by alcohol.

However, this medical equivalent of an infallible Papal Bull has been challenged from even within the profession. "The use of AAFs to estimate alcohol-related mortality … is questionable" says Professor Giovanni Corrao of Milan University, one of the world's top medical statisticians in the field of alcohol.[4]

Or put another way, you don't need a degree in logic to realise that merely asserting alcohol is related to certain conditions doesn't mean that they really are (by the way, if you are a logician, the fallacy is called *petitio principii* – in plain English, 'begging the question').

In fact, a cursory glance at the medical literature on so-called alcohol-related conditions reveals that it is shot through with *petitiones principii*. For example, here's what is widely acknowledged about the evidence for "Alcoholic Pancreatitis":

> The fact [is] that only a minority of less than 10% of heavy drinkers develop alcoholic pancreatitis.

– this from an authoritative 2010 paper by German alcohol experts.[5]

Or how about this statement on Alcoholic Liver Disease

(once again, completely supported by the clinical evidence), and its bold-as-brass oxymoronic conclusion:

> Only a small proportion of alcoholic patients develop advanced liver disease, suggesting that factors other than alcohol intake may influence Alcoholic Liver Disease.[6]

That comes from a 2012 paper in *Alcohol Clinical Experimental Research*, probably the field's most prestigious journal.

One view says that the only deaths which are unquestionably "alcohol-related" are those caused by alcoholism. Period.* That may sound a bit unsubtle, but although it's a minority view in 2013, it was actually the considered view of virtually the entire medical profession as recently as 1985.[7] Since then, the mortality statistics have confirmed that being an alcoholic shortens your life by about 20 years.[8]

However, over this same period, there has been what the military call "mission creep", where more and more "alcohol-related" diseases and deaths have been confidently promulgated, but often with scant scientific evidence, as we have seen in the last paragraphs.

There's a really simple solution to the alcohol-related disease issue, however. Since diseases tend to result in premature death, the easiest way to find out if alcohol is a disease risk is to ask a blunt, commonsense question: do drinkers die younger than non-drinkers?

You may be surprised to learn that there's a huge amount of evidence about alcohol and lifespan ... which you haven't heard about, of course, as it's a Good News story.

---

* Clearly, alcohol causes deaths due to accidents, car crashes, punch-ups, murder, suicides, etc, but I'm only dealing with alcohol and health here.

Living Doll

We all know that smoking causes lung cancer and other life-threatening diseases, but there was a time when we didn't. In the first half of the 20th century, when every film-star was a smoker (and many doctors too), most people thought cigs were not only harmless but even healthy.

The fact that we now find this belief ludicrous is down to some pioneering science in the 1950s. The driving force behind the work was a young British physician called Richard Doll, who was one of the first researchers in the then fledgling science of epidemiology (the study of a population's disease patterns and their possible causes).

Doll wanted to find out why lung cancer rates were increasing, so he decided to study a group of people he knew he'd get reliable data from – his fellow doctors. As I say, doctors were no different from the rest of the smoking population, and Doll did indeed find that most of his medic colleagues smoked, some getting through more than a pack of cigarettes a day.

He recruited about 35,000 doctors to the study and followed them for more than 4 years. What he discovered is now common knowledge: that there's a strong link between smoking and deaths from lung cancer, heart and respiratory disease. Central to his argument was the fact that there was a clear "dose response": the heaviest smokers had most disease, the lightest least.[9]

In recognition of his pioneering work, Doll was subsequently showered with honours, including a knighthood.

But why am I banging on about smoking in a book that's damn all to do with the subject? Because Professor Sir Richard Doll followed up his ground-breaking smoking study with an arguably even better one on alcohol.[10]

Doll began his alcohol study in 1978, again using doctors as his test-bed subjects. The design was simple: he first established how much each of them regularly drank, and then spent the next 13 years noting who died.

The doctors' average age at the start of the study was 62, so quite a few dropped dead during the study period. The graph overleaf shows the percentage of men who died, plotted against how much alcohol they regularly drank.

This is what Doll found:

Doctors' alcohol consumption & death rates

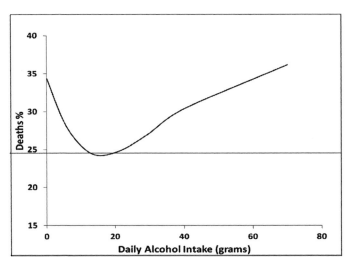

Derived from: Doll R et al. Mortality in relation to consumption of alcohol: 13 years' observations on male British doctors; *BMJ* 1994; 309: 91 1–8

First, let's look at the highest death rates. As you can see, most deaths occurred in two groups: 1. the men who drank the least, and 2. those who drank the most – about 70 grams a day.

This alone is an extraordinary finding. It says that drinking 70 grams of alcohol a day (a substantial amount, over twice the recommended maximum) is hardly more life-shortening than if you'd never touched a drop.

But the figures also reveal something equally remarkable: an inverse dose response. Unlike smoking, alcohol *reduces* death rates by a good 10%, albeit within certain intake levels.

And Doll's figures get even more interesting when you take into account the fact that quite a few of these deaths would have been caused by smoking. As his earlier study on smoking showed, many of his doctor subjects were smokers, and indeed Doll himself admits that there was "a close correlation between drinking and smoking habits". So could the death data have been skewed by the fact that drinkers also tend to be smokers?

Helpfully, Doll lists the precise causes of death of his doctor guinea-pigs, two of which are clearly smoking-related: lung cancer and respiratory disease. He also provides the actual number of deaths in each category, thus enabling one to re-analyse his data. So, what happens to the alcohol/mortality figures if we subtract the deaths caused by smoking?*

Doctors' daily alcohol consumption & death rates adjusted for smoking

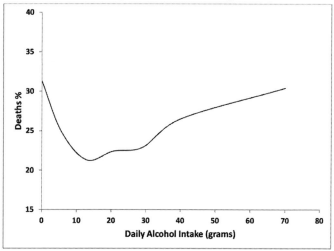

Derived from: Doll R et al. op. cit.

---

* This is scientifically perfectly respectable; it's called "adjusting for confounders".

Superficially, the graph doesn't look much different from before. But look closely, as there are two bombshell conclusions to be drawn from the reworked data.

First, the most life-shortening behaviour is to abstain from drinking. In other words, the primary cause of death among these men was the decision to be teetotal – not the decision to drink. The data showed that drinking even as much as 70 grams of alcohol a day was slightly less risky in terms of premature death than being teetotal.

Second, alcohol can reduce death rates by roughly 10%, a remarkable outcome achieved simply by drinking between about 15 and 30 grams of alcohol a day – ironically, almost the very amount we're told is the upper safe limit. Once again, as we've seen with heart disease, not drinking alcohol appears to be a major risk factor for premature death.

These extraordinary results were published in 1994, but what happened? Nothing.

Whereas Doll's 1956 ground-breaking findings on the dangers of smoking were to lead to a revolution in both medical thinking and public policy, the same didn't occur after his equally significant findings on the benefits of alcohol in extending lifespan. They have had not an iota of effect on medical thinking, which, as we are almost weekly reminded in the media, continues to insist that alcohol is dangerous to health. Very strange.

Of course, one reason why Doll's data was not acted upon could have been that they were a freak result. After all, medical science does occasionally throw up rogue findings which are later found to be wrong. But that's not possible in this case, because Doll's data has been amply confirmed by subsequent research.

In case you may be in any doubt about this, here are just a few long-term studies out of many that support his evidence.

1. "Late-life alcohol consumption and 20-year mortality"[11]
    When? 2010
    Where? USA (Stanford University, University of Texas,

Austin)

Who? 1800 "older adults"

How long? 20 years

Result: compared to people who drank up to 43 grams of alcohol a day, heavier drinkers had a 45% increase in death rate, but teetotallers even more: 51%.

Published conclusion:

> Even after taking into account traditional and non-traditional covariates, moderate alcohol consumption continued to show a beneficial effect in predicting mortality risk.

2. "Alcohol Consumption and All-Cause Mortality"[12]

When? 1995

Where? Whitehall & British Regional Heart Studies, UK

Who? 9000 middle-aged men

How long?: 7 to 10 years

Result: Minimum risk of death occurs at a consumption of about 31.5 grams of alcohol a day

Published conclusion:

> The 'sensible drinking level' of 21 units per week for men in the UK as a limit is not justified, and the data suggest that alcohol consumption is a net preventive factor against premature death.

3. "Alcohol Consumption and Mortality among Women"[13]

When? 1995

Where? Harvard University

Who? 85,000 female nurses

How long? 12 years

Results: Intakes of up to 5 grams of alcohol a day reduced death rates by 17%, and up to 30 grams a day by 12%.

Published conclusion:

> Light to moderate alcohol consumption is associated with a reduced mortality rate

4. "Type of Alcohol Consumed and Mortality from All Causes, Coronary Heart Disease, and Cancer"[14]

When? 2005

Where? University of Copenhagen

Who? 24,500 men & women aged 20-98

How long? 20 years

Results: People drinking beer and spirits (up to 36 grams of alcohol a day) had a maximum 10% reduction in death rates, but wine-drinkers had a maximum of 40% fewer deaths up to an intake over 60 grams a day.

Published conclusion:

> Wine intake may have a beneficial effect on all-cause mortality that is additive to that of alcohol. This effect may be attributable to a reduction in death from both coronary heart disease and cancer.

So here we have a total of five studies from across the world, all concluding the same thing: within certain intake limits, alcohol saves lives.

Some mistake surely

But common sense says that can't be true. After all, alcohol is a highly toxic substance. For example, if a 10 year old child were to drink a bottle of whisky, he would die within hours – and, of course, many alcoholics tend to suffer premature death, as we've already established.

Indeed, because doctors have found it hard to get their heads round the fact that the same substance might be both potentially lethal and life-extending, these lifespan studies initially caused lots of raised eyebrows.

The critics' major objection was that these were merely epidemiological studies, on disparate, uncontrolled populations, and thus it was impossible to be certain alcohol was the key factor in people's longevity. Never mind that these critics tended also to be the very same people who employed epidemiological data to claim alcohol causes all manner of diseases, but we'll let that pass.

The objection was perfectly respectable, however. As we've already seen in the Bad News chapter, epidemiology only allows you to claim "association" and not "causation". Remember the "smoking beagles" of the 1970s? They were sacrificed in order to test whether Doll's original lung cancer and tobacco association really was causal, even though everyone "knew" it had to be.*

So, what reasons have been put forward to question the validity of these 'alcohol extends lifespan' studies?

The issue turns around what are called "confounders" – things in people's lives that really have nothing to do with alcohol, but could throw up a spurious connection. The most obvious confounder is social class: wealthy people tend to drink a lot, but they also generally look after their health – by eating well, not smoking, exercising, affording medical care etc. Could that explain why drinkers appear to live longer? Not really. The social class explanation only washes if the people in the particular epidemiological survey come from widely differing income groups. But as we've already seen, two alcohol and longevity studies involved the same narrow social group: doctors in one study, nurses in another.

A more subtle confounder relates to why teetotallers choose not to drink. One suggestion put forward in the 1980s was that non-drinkers may be basically unwell – enough to put them off alcohol for life.[15] Or else, they may have already been drinkers but become teetotal because alcohol made them ill. If these so-called "sick quitters" were to form a substantial part of the teetotal group, that would unquestionably skew the longevity data in favour of alcohol.[16]

It turns out, however, that in practice this confounder is not much of a problem.

For example, the US researchers behind the study on 1800 people mentioned on page 104/5 tell us that they took great care to control for "former problem drinking status, existing health problems, and key socio-demographic and social-behavioural factors, as well as for age and gender," and found that this indeed "substantially reduced the mortality effect

---

* By the way, the dogs never got lung cancer from smoking – neither have rats, nor any other laboratory animals apart from mice ... and that took 40 years to demonstrate.

for abstainers compared to moderate drinkers." However, they were quick to point out that these confounders didn't alter the basic results:

> Even after adjusting for all covariates, abstainers ... continued to show increased mortality risks of 51% ... compared to moderate drinkers.[17]

To further test the sick quitter theory, a few studies have deliberately factored it in, and once again the overall outcomes aren't significantly affected. As a result, most experts now regard the sick quitter theory as a pretty dead duck.[18]

A final nail in the coffin for the sick quitter hypothesis is the evidence from alcohol's effect on already healthy people. For example, in their study on US male physicians, Harvard University researchers found that alcohol intake resulted in the same increase in extra health benefits – even among men who were already basically healthy.[19]

In case you might suspect that I'm picking cherry-picking the alcohol/mortality data, I'll come clean with you. Not every study shows that alcohol helps you live longer (not every study shows smoking causes lung cancer either) ... but, as I've said before, nothing is ever 100% reproducible in biology.[*]

Fortunately, however, medical statisticians have invented a way of deciding what's most likely to be true, even though there may be disparate findings between one research study and another. It's called meta-analysis, and it pools the data together, looking for general trends in the evidence. All a meta-analysis requires is enough raw data.

Is there enough alcohol and longevity data? You bet there is.

Over the years, as the evidence has gradually accumulated, a number of meta-analyses have been performed.

In 1996, Australian statisticians analysed the 16 long-term studies available at the time, and confirmed Doll's original findings. They calculated that maximum lifespan occurred at

---

[*]   Except for decapitation, exsanguination, suffocation, etc. which are invariably fatal.

a daily alcohol intake of 19 grams for men and 9 grams for women; the zero increase in death risk levels compared to non-drinkers were 39 grams for men and 28 grams for women.[20]

By 2006, the number of studies had risen to over 70, allowing a team of Italian statisticians to do a much more refined analysis – for example, being able to subdivide crude death rates into both gender and populations.[21]

Once again, the basic proposition that alcohol saves lives was validated, but European men were found to benefit most, followed by Americans and Asians. The sexes responded very differently too.

Here are two key graphs from that 2006 Italian paper:

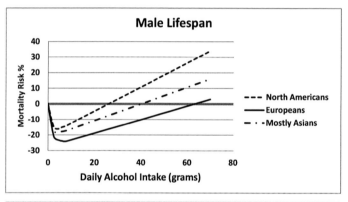

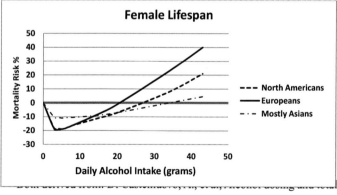

mortality in men and women: an updated meta-analysis of 34 prospective studies. *Arch Intern Med*. 2006 Dec 11–25; 166(22): 2437–45.

These graphs come from the combined data of about a million people all over the world, of whom 87,000 died during the periods of study. They overwhelmingly confirm that there is a J-shaped relationship between alcohol and death rates, i.e. that lower intakes reduce the mortality risk, while higher intakes increase it.

But alcohol's benefit differs markedly between both gender and population. At one extreme, European men seem to obtain the greatest benefit, with a maximum 22% reduction in risk of death, and the widest range of zero-risk intake: up to 67 grams of alcohol a day. By contrast, European women have slightly less longevity benefit and a much narrower zero-risk range, with a maximum super-safe intake of 22 grams a day. There are substantial differences between populations too: American men have the lowest benefits, as do Asian women – but the latter also have the widest female zero-risk range.

Why? The gender differences are easy to explain. After all, the sexes differ substantially in their biological response to alcohol – a subject we'll explore in the next chapter. But why the differences between populations?

The authors of the study admit to being a bit puzzled, but suggest two possible reasons: 1. Genes: Asians process alcohol differently from Europeans (Chapter 10 covers this in detail). 2. Different drinking patterns between USA and Europe: Europeans generally drink with meals, unlike Americans who tend to 'binge drink'.

To which I would add another possible explanation: because they eat less processed and more real food, continental Europeans are intrinsically healthier than Americans, so their bodies might be better at detoxifying alcohol.*

---

* By the way, the US figures are unlikely to have been affected by their African-American or Hispanic populations, whose alcohol-detoxifying genes are at least as good as Europeans'.

The Rodent Jury

For a final verdict on the whole issue of alcohol and lifespan, let's ask the opinion of our press-ganged animal jurists. In contrast to human beings, animals offer the cleanest, most clear-cut evidence, with no confounders of social class, sick quitters, feral youthful behaviour and the like.

Strangely, however, given medicine's predilection for animal experiments, only one study on alcohol and lifespan appears to have been undertaken. It was done way back in 1987, and it was a classic, fully controlled study on mice – and incidentally one in which the creatures might for once have had quite a nice time.[22] In addition to their normal feed, four identically housed groups of 100 mice were given either plain water, or water mixed with three different amounts of alcohol, corresponding to a low, moderate or "alcoholic" intake level for humans. Unusually for laboratory animals, the mice were allowed to die a natural death. What happened? Exactly the same as in the human studies: the mice that lived longest were the ones which drank "moderate" amounts of alcohol … every day for the whole of their adult lives.

So this huge body of research all points in the same direction: unless you go overboard on the booze, alcohol will help you live longer. In other words, the evidence is now overwhelming that alcohol in moderation saves lives.

Medical researchers have known this for decades, of course, so why haven't they told us? In writing this book, I've trawled through countless studies about the benefits of alcohol, and in 99.9% of them the conclusion boils down to either "these results should not be taken to suggest that people should start drinking", or "the most important public message is that excessive drinking is dangerous" – both of which mean the same thing: "for gawds sake don't tell them alcohol increases lifespan".

Which was the 0.1% of studies that dared to step out of line? Here's its conclusion:

> Heavy drinkers should be urged to cut their consumption,

but people who already regularly consume low to moderate amounts of alcohol should be encouraged to continue.

The authors weren't Americans, Brits, Swedes, Finns or Germans, who would never permit such a sentiment to pass their lips. So who wrote such subversive stuff? ... Italians – the statisticians whose study we covered at length on pages 108–110. [23]

So, please raise your glass and say in your best Italian accent:

"Salute; vita lunga e felicità!"
"Your good health; long life and happiness!"

10

Gender and Genes

One of the many reasons why life is so unfair is that we are largely stuck with the cards we've been dealt at birth. Two of the court cards in our hand are our gender and genes, and it turns out that both are hugely significant in how we respond to alcohol ... probably more than in any other field of health.

Which makes alcohol one of the unfairest things in life.

Women & Men

In this egalitarian era of ours, we tend to get twitchy about anything that highlights sex differences in any other areas than the obvious ones. But as we saw in the last chapter, alcohol is special: there are substantial health differences in the way that men and women respond to the liquid.

To recap, the evidence says that men can safely drink about twice as much alcohol as women.

That's a huge difference. There are no other autonomic bodily functions that are so different between the sexes – not energy needs, not oxygen requirements, not digestion ... nothing. In the realm of alcohol detoxification, it's as if men and women were different species.*

Why is alcohol so special? Why can men drink twice as much alcohol as women without coming to any harm whatever?

One reason often cited is that women are generally smaller than men and so have less body mass to absorb

---

* The politically incorrect might consider that a statement of the obvious.

114

the alcohol in. That explanation is OK as far as it goes, but women are only slightly smaller than men, not half their size. So that can't be the explanation. The theory has two variants, though: one says that women's bodies contain less water than men's, thus making it more difficult for them to dilute alcohol; the other says that because alcohol is not fat-soluble, and women's bodies contain more fat, *ergo* more alcohol ends up in female blood than men's.

But those arguments don't really wash either, because the amounts of body fat and water aren't that vastly different between the sexes.

There's got to be a more fundamental reason ... and there is, but you're going to have to stomach a bit of science.

As soon as you down a drink, your body immediately begins a detoxification process. In the stomach, where 20% of the alcohol is absorbed, there are digestive enzymes that try to break it down.

The remaining 80% goes through to the liver where another set of enzymes kick in.

So, before alcohol gets anywhere near the bloodstream (and thus before it can affect the brain or other organs), it first has to get processed by two sets of enzymes, both of which are specifically designed to detoxify alcohol. They have complicated scientific names, of course: alcohol dehydrogenase (ADH) and aldehyde dehydrogenase (ADLH).

Curiously, these are among the commonest enzymes on the planet – shared by not only human beings, but animals and even insects too. How come?

The prevailing theory is that alcohol-detoxifying enzymes evolved to allow all creatures to eat rotting fruit in safety.[1] This is not as far-fetched as it sounds: rotting fruit can contain up to 4% alcohol – a result of the chemical reaction between the fruit skin's natural yeasts and its juice.*

---

* I once had a flock of half a dozen chickens which used to scratch around beneath an apple tree in my garden. I vividly remember one late autumn day, when the ground was carpeted with windfall fruit, seeing the

It's these enzymes that are responsible for the sex differences.

The ADH enzymes are in charge of what's called "first-pass alcohol metabolism", where the alcohol is initially broken down. Here, there are fairly clear differences between the sexes, with women coming off worst, for the simple reason that they possess fewer of them – particularly women under the age of 40.[23]

The next (and principal) stage of alcohol processing happens in the liver where the ALDH enzymes kick in. It's these enzymes that do the vital detoxification of alcohol into harmless acetic acid. Sadly for women, they have far fewer of these enzymes too.[24]

So science says that women's inability to handle alcohol as efficiently as men is mainly due to having been dealt such a poor hand of alcohol-detoxifying enzymes. If you then add in the sex differences in body weight, water and fat, that ensemble could easily explain why women are so heavily on the boozing losing side.

This is strange. After all, over the millennia, most bodily functions and attributes have evolved in order to preserve the health of both sexes.

Why should women be so disfavoured? Frankly, I haven't a clue; I can't find anything in the scientific literature to explain it, either. All I can conclude is that, if the 'alcohol in rotting fruit' theory is correct, women's distant ancestors must have figured that it was damn stupid to eat rotten fruit, and much more sensible to pick fruit off the tree – durr!*

So women's inferior alcohol-detoxifying enzymes may be due to their superior intelligence.

But here comes another female fly in the ointment: the menopause. There is anecdotal evidence that women's unique marking of middle age also signals a significant change in

---

whole flock staggering around like a bunch of drunks on a Saturday night – all evidently made legless by the cider in the rotting apples.

* Isn't there a story about a lady called Eve who did just that with an apple?

their ability to handle alcohol.* Why? The medical literature says that, although the menopause doesn't affect ADH enzymes themselves, hormonal changes post-menopause may make women more intoxicated on smaller doses of alcohol. No-one knows how or why, however.[5]

But alcohol isn't only sexist and ageist, it's racist too.

Genes & Race

In the last chapter, we saw how Europeans tend to live longer than Asians, even when consuming the same amounts of alcohol. That's just one example of how alcohol is processed differently by different races.

Many of us are familiar with the stories of how European colonisation and its introduction of alcohol wiped out native populations – both cognitively and literally. Australia is one example,[6] the USA another.[7]

In both countries, alcoholism became rife among the indigenous populations. At first, the white man blamed it on fecklessness, but science has now begun to understand that there are cogent biological reasons for the "savages'" inability to hold their drink.

We now know that at least part of the problem is due to the fact that some non-Europeans lack crucial ADH and ALDH enzymes. This is entirely down to genetic inheritance, with the result that a substance which is fairly benign for Europeans becomes something more deadly for others. [8]

To those of us fortunate enough to enjoy alcohol's mental effects, it's perhaps worth reminding ourselves just how poisonous alcohol – i.e fermented fruit juice (wine and cider), fermented grains (beer) and their distilled derivatives (spirits) – really can be.

Think of what alcohol is used for when it's not glugging down our throats.

---

* A fact confirmed by many of my female friends *d'un certain age,* whose dinner party glasses need less refilling as the years go by.

Alcohol (and its identical partner, ethanol) is an important industrial chemical, being used both as a powerful solvent and as an additive to petrol – indeed, cars will run entirely on ethanol.

Alcohol is also a potent disinfectant, routinely used by hospitals as a hand-cleanser to prevent infection. To borrow the familiar script of lavatory cleaner commercials, alcohol kills 99.9% of germs stone dead. So it's as vicious as bleach.

It's also a powerful preservative. If you want to keep a corpse (or any parts thereof) from rotting, immerse it in alcohol. It will last for ever. Only formalin will do as good a job.

So alcohol is seriously cytotoxic – it kills living cells.

The puzzle is therefore not why indigenous Australians and Americans go crazy on alcohol, but why Europeans don't. After all, if we Europeans were to drink formalin or bleach, it would send us crazy too … before killing us. In principle alcohol is no different.

What's so special about booze? Why are most of us resistant to its poisonous effects?

One explanation we've already mentioned is the rotting fruit theory. But that can't be the whole story. After all, we humans would have given up eating rotten fruit thousands of years ago when we became farmers.

And that's the clue. When humans developed agriculture, we became settled, ceasing to become nomadic hunter-gatherers, and – crucially – losing access to pure water. For, along with settlements came the inevitable downsides of crowding together, one of which is a lack of sanitation.

At some stage, the settled communities would have noticed that some people got ill or even died after drinking the communal water, but that others didn't – and that the difference between the two groups was that the survivors added fermented juice from fruit or grains to their water, in preference to drinking plain water.

Whether our farming ancestors 12,000 years ago knew that alcohol was the equivalent of today's water-purifying chlorine is not recorded. However, we do know that by the time of the Ancient Greeks and Romans, wine was often drunk admixed with water, thus offering a disinfected source of vital H2O.

By the medieval period, as Northern Europe's climate cooled, wine gave way to ale and mead as the drink of the common people, who tended to drink these in preference to water. Once again, this meant that people's liquid intake would have been fully disinfected.

Although medieval ale and mead had a fairly low alcoholic content, and were possibly further diluted with water, everyone must have been going around mildly sloshed, and thus laden with a good deal of alcohol to detoxify every day. In Elizabethan England, for example, historian Ian Mortimer tells us that "the daily allowance for a man – whether he be a servant or a nobleman – in many large houses [was] a gallon of beer, and this is not a notional amount: people really [did] drink that much on a regular basis".[9] So there would have been powerful evolutionary selection pressures favouring those people who possessed the alcohol-detoxifying enzymes inherited from their rotten fruit-eating forebears. Quite simply, the people who lacked the enzymes would have found alcohol made them feel ill, and would have shunned it … with possibly fatal consequences. Thus, the winners in the survival and subsequent breeding stakes would have been the people genetically lucky enough to have the right AHD and ADLH enzymes.

So it is the need to sanitise drinking water which may explain why Europeans (and those of European ancestry) have such a robust complement of these alcohol-defying enzymes. This is likely to be the primary explanation for the racial differences in the alcohol/longevity stakes we saw in the last chapter, with European men far outstripping everyone else.

How do other races fare, enzyme-wise?

Perhaps surprisingly, the least favoured ethnic groups turn out to be not Australian and American natives but Asian Mongoloids (Japanese, Chinese, and South-East Asians) and a few South American tribes.[10]

The most obvious effect of these populations' lack of alcohol-detoxifying enzymes is a visual one: their faces flush a deep red when they drink even "the amounts of alcohol that have no detectable effects on Europeans".[11] The flushing is believed to be caused by acetaldehyde, the first breakdown product of alcohol. As we saw in Chapter 2, acetaldehyde is the poisonous intermediate step in the process by which the body detoxifies alcohol. In Europeans, ADLH enzymes quickly convert acetaldehyde to harmless acetic acid, but this fairy godmother's magic wand is genetically denied to about 50% of Asians; their lack of the right genes means that the conversion to acetic acid is seriously delayed.[12]

As it's a poison, acetaldehyde makes one feel pretty ropey, so it's no surprise that many Asians tend to shun alcohol.[13]

What about other races?

Perhaps surprisingly, there are no genetic examples quite as cut and dried as the Asian one. In fact, there is quite a lot of, in the jargon, "linkage disequilibrium and diversity" – a posh term for the fact that worldwide the alcohol detoxing genes are a bit of a jumble.[14]

So it's difficult to say anything very conclusive about race and genes, other than the simple point that Europeans are generally the most favoured.

However, even within this favoured group, there are some important and unfortunate exceptions – among them the people who, in the medical jargon, become "dependent" … in other words, addicts.

Genes & Alcoholics

The main reason why genes and alcohol are such a hot medical topic is not for racial research, but to try and explain why some drinkers become alcoholics, while the vast majority don't. The figures vary, with authoritative estimates of the number of people becoming alcoholics ranging between 5-10 % of normal drinkers – partly because of differences in defining who's an alcoholic. We'll cover alcoholism in the next chapter, but here we'll focus on genetics.

Genes are thought to be important because alcoholism tends to run in families. It was once thought that children growing up in a boozing household merely aped their parents' behaviour. But medics are now certain that can't be the whole story, because twins born to alcoholics, if separated in early childhood, share an increased risk of becoming "dependent", no matter what their upbringing.[15]

So it's thought that alcoholism must be at least in part genetically determined.

However, the search for the rogue gene or genes which can turn mere "social" drinkers into "dependent" ones has been rather frustrating ... but it's not been for want of trying.

In 1989, eight leading US research centres collaborated in an intensive genetic mapping of over 11,000 American alcoholics. The first thing they confirmed was the familial connection, showing that roughly half the risk of becoming alcoholic was down to whether the parents were alcoholics. Initially researchers were pretty confident they'd find the gene or genes responsible. But decades on, not much progress has been made: it's still unclear which specific genes are really responsible for alcoholism. The best that modern research can come up with is that some variants of one or two alcohol-detoxifying genes may be important, but "exactly how these variants affect alcohol metabolism remains to be discovered", the researchers admit.[16]

A few other genes have been implicated, but they tend to be related to behavioural traits (such as impulsivity) rather than to alcohol enzymes themselves.

So, after nearly 30 years research, science has yet to come up with a cogent explanation of alcoholism – or as two of the leading researchers so elegantly expressed it:

> Alcoholism is genetically complex, meaning that multiple genes are likely to be involved, and their interactions with one another and with an individual's environment also have to be examined before a complete picture of the processes that can lead to the disorder is assembled.[17]

– in other words, as far as alcoholism and genes are concerned, we haven't the foggiest.

Genes & Normal Drinkers

Chapter 2 mentioned an in-depth Italian study which announced the medically heretical discovery that most drinkers – even heavy ones – had no health problems with alcohol whatsoever. Puzzled by the findings, the physicians asked their geneticist colleagues to investigate, and they found that the people who had a problem with high intakes of alcohol also had an uncommon "allele" (variant) of an ALDH gene, the one responsible for the chief set of protective enzymes.[18]

Once that discovery had occurred, similar findings poured in from all over the world. It was soon found that the risk of getting cirrhosis of the liver also depends on whether you've got one of the right ALDH variants.[19]

On the plus side, another variant has been found to be best at protecting you from a heart attack.[20]

In Asians, two variants of the ALDH2 gene have been found to result in substantial disparities in the speed of clearing the blood of acetaldehyde, alcohol's poisonous by-product – producing major differences in facial flushing, heart rate and even "psychomotor performance", thus affecting driving skills.[21]

The study of genetics and alcohol is still in it infancy, but these are interesting and promising first steps. Just as the pharmaceutical industry has come to recognise that genetic differences explain why we don't all react to drugs and medications in the same way, physicians may soon be able to appreciate that a "one size fits all" approach is inappropriate for alcohol too.

Given that most of the human race (apart from Asians) seem to have the right protective genes to combat alcohol toxicity, science needs merely to advance sufficiently to be able to identify which of us may have the rogue genetic variants, and tailor individual health advice accordingly.

But that day appears to be some way off.

11

Avoiding Alcoholism

Of all the health hazards of alcohol, becoming addicted is far and away the most damaging. The Good News, however, is that most of us won't become alcoholics – although medics try to scare us rigid by suggesting otherwise.

How many drinkers actually become alcoholics is a matter of dispute, though. Some experts say it's only tiny minority, but others claim it's a substantial number of drinkers who are –in the jargon – "dependent" on alcohol.

I put the word dependent in quotes because it's what medics call those whom they think have "an alcohol problem". However, people whom some experts claim are likely to be alcohol-dependent don't really fit the layman's image of the typical alcoholic.

For example, one theory says that you may be "dependent" if you drink every day – however little … which is one reason why medics encourage us to lay off the drink for a couple of days a week.

Sensible ordinary folk don't really need to have the obvious objections spelt out, but I will anyway, for the benefit of my medic readers:

1. By this 'one drink-a-day' definition, virtually the entire adult populations of France, Italy and Spain are on Skid Row.

2. Condemning a voluntary activity simply because one performs it daily is silly. For example, I feel the need to brush my teeth at least once day, and would probably suffer mild withdrawal symptoms if I didn't. Thus, I'm a tooth-brushing addict, but so what? The issue is whether my behaviour is harmful, not how often I perform it, and as we've seen, alcohol is largely beneficial below substantial intakes.

3. Many alcoholics in treatment have repeated cycles of days of total abstinence followed by days of uncontrolled drinking. Therefore, according to the drink-a-day definition, these people are not dependent on alcohol.

Fortunately, however, medical science has come up with a more rational definition of alcoholism. It's to be found in the "DSM IV Criteria"[1] – a reference manual used by psychiatrists the world over.* The manual defines alcoholism as "A maladaptive pattern of alcohol use, leading to clinically significant impairment or distress." I won't quote any more, as it's far too expensive to obtain the reprinting rights, but in summary the manual says that if your behaviour ticks at least three of the following boxes, you're an addict:

1. You need more and more drink to get drunk.

2. Paradoxically, you need less and less drink to get drunk.

3. You get withdrawal symptoms, making you reach for more booze (or drugs like valium) to cure them.

4. You keep on drinking more than you really mean to.

5. You keep on trying to cut down, but fail.

6. You spend an awful lot of time in the whole booze game: getting the stuff, drinking it, and then recovering from its effects.

7. Your life outside the home suffers: you don't socialise any more, work gets difficult, and you stop having fun.

8. You keep on drinking even when you know it's causing physical or mental problems, such as a stomach ulcer or depression.

To which I would suggest one more:

9. You lie about how much you drink and try and hide the evidence.

Many of us will be able to recognise those characteristics in people we know. But, unless you're reading this on a park bench amidst a sea of empty cider tinnies, I bet only a small percentage of your drinking friends are so afflicted. For the

---

* There is an updated DSM-V version, but it has been widely criticised for its lack of commonsense and implicit pandering to Big Pharma.

plain fact is that the vast majority of drinkers never become alcoholics by the DSM-IV definition ... however much they drink.

So the real question is this: what is it about alcoholics that makes them so different?

As we saw in the last chapter, the answer is only possibly genetic. After all, if it were totally to do with inheritance, 30 years of research would surely have identified the rogue genes by now.

Thus, if alcoholism is only partly due to nature, its major cause must be some combination of nurture, environment, personality and poor lifestyle choices.

What might these be?

I'll have a stab at an answer. After all, a book that says that having more than a drink a day is good for your health, also has a duty to help you avoid having too much of a good thing.

First, let's see what advice doctors give.

As we saw in Chapter 9, becoming seriously addicted to alcohol can shorten your life by about 20 years. That's a serious medical problem, so you'd expect there to be a plethora of official advice about how to avoid becoming an alcoholic.

There isn't.

I've spent days searching diligently within the obvious official sources of information from Britain's health bodies such as the NHS and Dept of Health. But there's nothing. Their leaflets and web pages are full of the usual stuff about the dangers of drinking more than the sacrosanct standard 21 units a week. But they say nothing about how to prevent alcoholism.

"You're obviously looking in the wrong places, you idiot", I told myself. "Why not check with the Press Offices?"

Because official bodies are hungry for publicity, they employ small armies of "communications officers", whose main job is to make life easy for journalists by feeding them their employers' Public Relations messages on a plate.

So I began a little email journey down what I imagined would be corridors of open doors.

First, the Dept of Health's Press Officer with special responsibility for drugs and alcohol.

"Hi xxx", I emailed, *"I'm a freelance hack currently researching alcohol & health. I'm looking for any docs containing official (NHS/DoH etc) advice on how to prevent alcoholism/avoid becoming an alcoholic. I'm obviously being stoooopid* (attempt at levity) *but I can't find anything on any UK govt website. Can you help me out please? Many thanks, Tony Edwards"*

But answer came there none. I then tried his boss, who replied: *"I will be out of the office (blah blah) ... I will reply on my return"*. She didn't.

OK, I thought, if officialdom can't help with advice on preventing alcoholism, surely the alcohol charities will. After all, a bit like government, they're funded by the taxpayer, because their supporters get tax relief on their donations.

Start at the top, I thought: Alcoholics Anonymous. However, I searched their website but found nothing relevant. OK, same email sent to AA's press office. Within an hour I got this reply:

> Dear Tony,
>
> Thank you for your email seeking information on prevention of alcoholism. We in Alcoholics Anonymous are here solely to help those with a serious alcohol problem achieve and maintain sobriety. Our AA Tradition tells us we ought not to become involved in debate on alcohol levels nor hold an opinion on any outside issues. For information on safe levels of alcohol or prevention of damage an organization such as Alcohol Concern may prove helpful. Thank you once again for your inquiry.

Somewhat stunned, I replied: *"Thanks. So ... just to confirm: can I say that AA gives no advice on how to prevent people needing their help? Regards, Tony E."* Answer: none.

However, AA had mentioned Alcohol Concern, another

charity. So I bunged them the same pleading email.

Quick as a flash, Alcohol Concern's Press Officer penned this:

> Hi Tony
>
> We're not an alcohol service provider, meaning that we don't see or counsel people who have or think they might have a problem so we don't have a lot of material around that.
>
> We'd say there are things we can do to make sure the reduce the harm caused by alcohol, so for instance we campaign for a minimum unit price, we've done research into connections between gambling and alcohol, looked at off licence outlet density (so the connection between alcohol related problems and alcohol availability).
>
> If you're looking for that more medical angle it's a good idea to get in touch with a service provider, perhaps Foundation 66 or Phoenix Futures or I can send you some more info on some of our campaigning areas.
>
> Cheers, [*sic!*]
> [name]

So I tried the two charities suggested by Alcohol Concern. Here's the email I got from Foundation 66:

> Hi Tony
>
> This may help http://www.alcoholconcern.org.uk/concerned-about-alcohol.[*]
>
> This is also a good test https://dontbottleitup.org.uk/[†] Essentially, people should try to stick within the safe drinking guidelines:
>
> - men should not regularly drink more than three to four units of alcohol per day
> - women should not regularly drink more than two to three units of alcohol per day
> - you should take a break for 48-hours after a heavy

---

[*]   Yes, the very same Alcohol Concern

[†]   This is quite fun to do, actually

drinking session to let your body recover.

The signs that people may be developing a problem with alcohol come when someone feels that they 'need' alcohol to have a good time, feel confident, relax etc. If you are craving an alcoholic drink during the day or when at work, then you would be seen as at a high risk of developing problem drinking.

Most GPs have had training in supporting people who may have problems with alcohol and many can refer people very quickly to on-site on local advice and support – wc call that 'brief interventions'. We would recommend that people talk to their GP about their concerns openly and honestly.

Most boroughs/councils have at least one type of alcohol 'drop in' centre, like this http://www.foundation66.org.uk/pages/alcoholresourcecentre.html

It's worth checking on your local authority website.

Here's the reply from Phoenix Futures:

Hi Tony,

We don't currently provide that information on our website. For your research, you may want to contact Alcohol Concern, website address: http://www.alcoholconcern.org.uk/ and/ or look on the Talk To Frank website http://www.talktofrank.com/

Phoenix Futures is a service provider for people with drug, alcohol and gambling problems and we want someone needing help to contact us directly so that we can look at different treatment options available to them.

So ... the parcel having been comprehensively passed in my native land, I pinged an email across the pond to America's National Institute on Alcohol Abuse and Alcoholism. Being a mere freelance hack and a Limey to boot, I didn't expect much joy there either, but back came this:

Hi Tony.

Here are some ideas to get you started:

Rethinking Drinking -- http://rethinkingdrinking.

niaaa.nih.gov/ -- a NIAAA website designed to help people reduce their risk for alcohol problems.

Preventing Alcohol Abuse and Alcoholism—An Update (an issue of Alcohol Research & Health, NIAAA's peer-reviewed, scientific journal). Available at: http://pubs.niaaa.nih.gov/publications/arh342/toc34_2.htm

I would also suggest you peruse our brochures and fact sheets at: http://www.niaaa.nih.gov/publications/brochures-and-fact-sheets, as well as our Clinician's Guide:

http://pubs.niaaa.nih.gov/publications/Practitioner/CliniciansGuide2005/clinicians_guide.htm

I hope these materials are useful. Please let me know if you need more information or have additional questions.

Best regards,
John Bowersox

Press Office
National Institute on Alcohol Abuse and Alcoholism
5635 Fishers Lane, Room 3101, Bethesda,
MD 20892-9304

So, bless his cotton sox, here's a flavour of the advice John Bowersox at NIAAA generously offers anyone worried about becoming an alcoholic:

Here are some strategies to try, and you can add your own at the end. Check off perhaps two or three to try in the next week or two.

1 Keep track. Keep track of how much you drink. Find a way that works for you, carry drinking tracker cards in your wallet, make check marks on a kitchen calendar, or enter notes in a mobile phone notepad or personal digital assistant. Making note of each drink before you drink it may help you slow down when needed.

2 Count and measure. Know the standard drink sizes so you can count your drinks accurately. Measure drinks at home. Away from home, it can be hard to keep track, especially with mixed drinks, and at times, you may be getting more alcohol than you think. With wine, you may need to ask the host or server not to "top off" a partially filled glass.

3 Set goals. Decide how many days a week you want to drink and how many drinks you'll have on those days. It's a good idea to have some days when you don't drink. Drinkers with the lowest rates of alcohol use disorders stay within the low-risk limits.

4 Pace and space. When you do drink, pace yourself. Sip slowly. Have no more than one standard drink with alcohol per hour. Have "drink spacers"—make every other drink a non-alcoholic one, such as water, soda, or juice.

5 Include food. Don't drink on an empty stomach. Eat some food so the alcohol will be absorbed into your system more slowly.

6 Find alternatives. If drinking has occupied a lot of your time, then fill free time by developing new, healthy activities, hobbies, and relationships, or renewing ones you've missed. If you have counted on alcohol to be more comfortable in social situations, manage moods, or cope with problems, then seek other, healthy ways to deal with those areas of your life.

7 Avoid "triggers." What triggers your urge to drink? If certain people or places make you drink even when you don't want to, try to avoid them. If certain activities, times of day, or feelings trigger the urge, plan something else to do instead of drinking. If drinking at home is a problem, keep little or no alcohol there.

8 Plan to handle urges. When you cannot avoid a trigger and an urge hits, consider these options: Remind yourself of your reasons for changing (it can help to carry them in writing or store them in an electronic message you can access easily). Or talk things through with someone you trust. Or get involved with a healthy, distracting activity, such as physical exercise or a hobby that doesn't involve drinking. Or, instead of fighting the feeling, accept it and ride it out without giving in, knowing that it will soon crest like a wave and pass. Also, see the short module to help you handle urges to drink.

9 Know your "no." You're likely to be offered a drink at times when you don't want one. Have a polite, convincing "no, thanks" ready. The faster you can say no to these offers, the less likely you are to give in. If you hesitate, it allows you time to think of excuses to go along. Also, see the short module to help you build drink refusal skills.

John is clearly intelligent enough to realise that these are unlikely to have universal appeal (particularly to non-folksy Europeans), but they're sensible, and pretty well the best on offer.

Why is there such a dearth of official advice about how to avoid descending into the hell of alcoholism? Two reasons perhaps. First, nobody has a much of a clue why only some people succumb, and second (astonishingly for all their talk about the dangers of the demon drink), there's been little effort to research effective preventive strategies. The authorities are content simply to repeat the standard mantra: "don't drink more than 21 units a week". But that's clearly far too lame.

There is one strategy that has been tried, which appears to be the best they can up with is. What is it? … wait for it … it's getting a pep talk from your GP. I kid you not.* That's not what it's called, of course; the official medic-speak term for GP finger-wagging is "Screening and Brief Intervention" (SBI).

A 2012 survey describes SBI as:

> Brief structured advice typically employed in time-limited situations, such as general medical practice, with immediate intervention following screening. The intervention typically lasts between 5 and 10 minutes and usually consists of a standard package involving information on drinking risk levels, the status of the patient's own drinking in relation to those levels, encouragement to cut down and set a date for doing so, and a few simple hints on how cutting down might best be achieved, often accompanied by self-help material.[2]

---

* Ironically, one of the (admittedly tongue-in-cheek) definitions of being an alcoholic is "drinking more than your GP."

Sounds OK as far as it goes, but although SBI has been tried enthusiastically in a few heavy-drinking countries, surprise surprise it's been largely a failure. A 2012 report assessed a quarter of a century's experience and had to conclude: "There is a need for evidence that SBI results in reductions to alcohol-related mortality and morbidity"[3] – in other words, SBI doesn't work.

Another group of medics who have got involved in alcoholism are psychiatrists, who say they've identified a particular personality characteristic: a tendency to behave impulsively. Also, again surprise surprise, there's often a background of depression.

With the development of brain imaging technology, there's been quite a lot of research on alcoholics' actual brain processes. MRI scans tend to show characteristic patterns of brain "excitation exceeding and overpowering inhibition in the alcoholic subjects' brains.", says an expert US research report.[4]

> This imbalance, or "disinhibition," can also be seen in the children of alcoholics and strongly predicts their own subsequent development of heavy drinking and alcohol dependence, which suggests that these patterns are a marker for a biologically inherited predisposition to alcoholism.

So, no marks for guessing that, faced with such powerful events in the brain, conventional psychiatry finds alcoholism a pretty tough nut to crack.

What else is on offer?

Predictably, the pharmaceutical companies have got in on the act, and that's where most of the medical research has been focused (as ever, follow the money).

But despite their mighty brains and even mightier cheque books, the drug companies have struggled to find anything that reliably helps the alcoholism-prone drinker. That's rather surprising, as literally thousands of rats have paid with their lives to demonstrate that there are four or five key brain chemicals involved with alcohol addiction (if you must know, mainly dopamine, serotonin, opioids such as endorphins, and glutamate). So you'd think that finding substances to "antagonise" these chemicals and so cure alcoholism would be a doddle.

Indeed, that's what the drug companies initially expected, but that hope has since largely turned to dust. Yes, they've found the correct "antagonist drugs", but they don't reliably work.[5]

Some alcoholics do indeed respond to some drugs, but the benefits are nothing dramatic, and doctors find it impossible to predict who's going to benefit from which drug anyway. In fact, they've had to admit that a whole decade's worth of intensive research has been "disappointing", [6] explaining that:

> Heterogeneity in treatment response makes it necessary
> to characterize genetic and protein markers and endo-
> phenotypes for individualized pharmacotherapy".*

In other words, because the drugs are so hit and miss, science is going to have to discover much more about people's individual differences in order to come up with some really targeted alcoholism drugs.

Anything else on offer?

As far as I can see, nothing. In terms of expert advice and help preventing alcoholism … er … that appears to be it.

DIY Alcoholism Prevention

So, given such a paltry choice of successful evidence-based prevention strategies, let me suggest a few of my own. As with many of the official ones, they're also without supporting clinical evidence, but so what? They can't be much worse than the stuff already on offer.

---

* See what ghastly prose I've had to plough through to bring you the facts!

So, here are some extra, ***totally untested*** (some obviously tongue-in-cheek) ideas on how to avoid becoming an alcoholic.

1. Don't drink before 6 pm

Many drinkers know this from long experience, of course. Lunchtime drinking may give you a temporary lift, but at the price of feeling seedy all day; whereas the same amount of alcohol drunk in the evening has the opposite effect.

To the '6pm rule', some drinkers jauntily riposte: "it's 6pm somewhere in the world" (ha bloody ha). But it's not clock time that's important, it's 'body clock' time. Here's the explanation.

Nature has cleverly arranged things so that all life forms – plants, animals and humans – respond to the changing time of day. Over the millennia, we've all developed what are called circadian rhythms. These are fluctuations in the body's various systems to prepare them to be active at the appropriate time of day. They go through a whole cycle roughly every 24 hours (Latin: circa=about, dies=day). For example, at about 4 am, there are changes in the levels of hormone melatonin in order to help us wake up.

There are also circadian rhythms in the enzymes that detoxify alcohol. These follow a regular daily peak and trough cycle. As a result, the human body finds it more difficult to process alcohol in the morning, so that the same amount of booze will squirt 30% more alcohol into the blood in the morning than the evening – and twice as fast, too.[7]

Why this should be so, nobody really knows – although I'll hazard a guess that it's Nature's way of ensuring we don't slack on the hunting and gathering, finally rewarding us with a convivial booze-up after the day's toil.[*]

I would have thought that the fact that alcohol metabolism is dramatically different at different times of the day might

---

[*] On the other hand, rats also show exactly the same daily variation; decide for yourself if this supports my little theory.

be a crucial piece of health information. But I've searched the "alcohol is Bad News" propaganda, and found scarcely a mention of it.

But it could be important. Let me tell you a story about a friend of mine.

I'll call her Sally. Because she was married to a successful adman, she didn't need to work. One morning while doing the ironing, she felt bored. She wondered what it would be like … to have a gin & tonic – only a little one, mind you … Oooh! Nice feeling; boredom gone; let's have another. You can guess the rest; it was a modern Rake's Progress.

She continued the post-breakfast drinking for weeks, and one fine day, while out shopping in the car, she had a minor prang. People smelt alcohol on her breath, and she was bang to rights: 12 month driving ban. Now housebound, she became even more bored, and so stepped up the drinking. Within a few months, she had become a raging alcoholic. She was once seen by friends to vomit blood in the loo and then nonchalantly pour herself another vodka. One afternoon, two of her girl friends dropped in uninvited, and found her in bed choking on her own vomit. Were it not for that chance visit, she might well have died.

There's a happy ending, though. Sally did a course of group therapy for alcoholics, and was 99% cured – the missing 1% being the fact that she can't ever touch a drop again. That's sad. She's a very attractive, sociable woman who now gets discomfited by dinner parties because she can't really join in the merriment. And of course, by being a teetotaller she's shortening her life.

But the real moral of the story is that it's conceivable she might not have become an alcoholic if she'd known that Nature dictates that morning drinking is a Really Bad Idea.*

As an interesting aside, after Sally was rushed to hospital at the height of her addiction, her liver was found to be 100% normal.

---

* One sign of alcoholism is morning drinking – but of course that doesn't mean much, as which came first: the morning drinking or the addiction?

2. Don't drink when depressed

If you're suffering from depression, don't use drink to cure it.

I'm talking about all kinds of depression – from feeling down in the dumps to really severe so-called "clinical" depression. Writer Marian Keyes, depressive and former alcoholic, says clinical depression is like "living in hell".[8]

If you're already living in hell, don't drink, use anti-depressants;[*] drink will only get you out of hell via a coffin.

If you're merely down in the dumps, alcohol won't make it any better, and you run the risk of going from the frying pan into the fire.

That said, there is some evidence that careful drinking may actually reduce the risk of getting depression in the first place, with wine appearing especially beneficial. But that's only up to intakes of about 15 grams a day.[9]

Heavy drinking, however, unquestionably increases the risk of major depression.[10]

3. Self-inflicted aversion therapy

I offer this technique because it's how I made myself quit smoking (I was a "pack a day" man well into my 30s); however, let me stress I have absolutely no idea if it would work with booze.

With cigarettes, I waited until I got a severe cold and then forced myself to chain-smoke, inhaling deeply. Really grisly. Never smoked again.[†]

I've been trying figure out what the booze equivalent might be – but please don't take any of this too seriously!

1. Wait until you've got a stomach bug and then glug lots of cheap plonk.[‡]

---

[*] Contrary to press reports, these do work, but only in genuine clinical depression.

[†] Except the very occasional cadged one – thanks, folks! It means I'm 100% cured, though.

[‡] Actually there's some evidence this might cure the stomach bug (see Chapter 12)

2. Twirl yourself round and round for 10 seconds until you're giddy, take a slurp of neat gin, then carry on twirling. Repeat until you collapse in a pseudo-drunken heap.

3a. Take a weekend break to any low-rent British city centre, and after midnight closely inspect the randomly deposited stomach and bladder contents.

3b. Ditto ... observe the behaviour of your fellow human [question mark] beings.

4. Is it just the taste I'm after?

Interrogate your taste buds before pouring a drink. Is it really the alcohol hit they need, or would a strong-tasting drink like fruit juice do just as well instead?

5. Get yourself genetically tested – after 2020

This one is really no more than a hope. I say 2020, because if you're reading this book then, science may have advanced sufficiently to have discovered why some drinkers become alcoholics but others don't. The answer will probably have to come from genetics, but, as we saw in the Gender & Genes chapter, at present the science is too flimsy.

Lest I get sued for dishing out dodgy advice, let me reiterate that these are all totally untested suggestions about how to avoid social drinking morphing into addiction. They are completely without any supporting medical evidence. Nos 1, 2 and 4 and 5 will of course do no harm at all, but if you totally lack a sense of humour, you attempt No 3's little suggestions entirely at your own risk.

Nuff said.

About time we had some more Good News ...

To recap. As we've already explored exhaustively from Chapter 2 onwards, alcohol is good for your health, preventing heart disease, dementia, diabetes, arthritis, some cancers, etc. etc. But alcohol isn't one liquid: it comes in different types, of course. We humans have been quite canny in creating a range of alcoholic drinks with distinct flavours – each geared for different situations. For example, only a cold beer or white wine will satisfy on a sunny day, red wine is best with a heavy dinner, and spirits and fortified wines are *comme il faut* before or after meals as aperitifs or digestifs.

The question is this: do any of these drinks have any *extra* health benefits over and above the alcohol content itself? In other words, can the Good News get Even Better?

In the next three chapters we'll explore the individual health merits of the three main alcohol types: wine, beer and spirits. The first chapter is VERY long, the second is the reverse, and the third is probably the shortest chapter ever written in publishing history.

12

Even Better News about Wine

Let's skip the bog-standard intro: "Wine was first fermented in … by the …, and has been a staple alcoholic drink for …", and get straight down to the extra Good News about wine and health.

There's oodles of it, but sadly for lovers of Pinot Grigio, Sauvignon, Chardonnay etc., the Even Better News applies mainly to red wine.

Happily, science has a pretty good idea why red wine is so beneficial to health, which gives us confidence that the connection between red wine and good health may be genuinely causal, rather than a mere association, which is the basic problem with most of the alcohol/health research.

I'll cover the chemistry of wine later in this chapter, but first let's look at the actual health evidence. Earlier chapters have covered some of it, but here's a pull-together of the medical data, disease by disease.

Breast Cancer
Chapter 2 mentioned a study done in 2008 on about 1500 women in Southern France.[1] The authors, Professors Faiza Bessaoud and Jean-Pierre Daurès, were two of France's top "biostatisticians", both working for INSERM, the French equivalent of Britain's Medical Research Council. They chose the Hérault area "where wine is an integral part of the population's dietary habits", and identified every woman – young and old – who was diagnosed with breast cancer over a two-year period. These women's entire lifestyles were then analysed in detail, including the types of alcohol they drank, how much and how often. Another matched 'control

group' of healthy women without breast cancer was similarly surveyed.

The findings were dramatic. First, none of the breast cancer cases appeared to have any association with alcohol intake – no matter how much nor what type of alcohol the women drank. As an aside, the single most important lifestyle factor connected with breast cancer was "high consumption of red meat" (roughly doubling the cancer risk). Second, up to an intake of 15 grams of alcohol a day, wine *reduced the risk* of breast cancer – by a remarkable 42%. Third, the greatest protection occurred among the women who drank wine every day; there was no benefit whatever if their intake was "sporadic". Fourth, higher intakes of wine did not increase cancer risk at all.

So the researchers had no option but politely to stick two fingers up to their Anglo-Saxon prohibitionist colleagues, and conclude that:

> Low and regular consumption of wine reduces the risk of breast cancer. … It is [therefore] perhaps not suitable to advise that all low alcohol consumers, especially wine drinkers, reduce their alcohol intake.

Two years later those French findings were bolstered by some somewhat less dramatic results in a Canadian study on pre-menopausal women.[2]

> Compared to non-drinkers, exclusive consumption of wine was associated with a significant reduction in the risk of breast cancer

reported the 20-strong Hereditary Breast Cancer Group at the University of Ottawa. However, the effect was confined to one particular breast cancer type – the relatively rare BRCA1 genetic mutation.

What makes these 'wine prevents breast cancer' results even more interesting and credible are three pioneering research studies from the USA. The first was published in 1998 by scientists at the hugely prestigious Mayo Clinic, who made the remarkable discovery that red wine appears to have some very healthy effects on actual breast tissue. This was discovered almost by chance in a long-term dietary survey of about 1500 women who were also undergoing routine mammography (breast cancer diagnosis by X-Ray). One of the survey's breast checks involved measuring the density of the breasts, as this is a known risk factor for breast cancer: the denser the breast tissue, the greater risk of cancer – up to 5 times higher.[3]

The researchers were surprised to stumble on a connection between breast density and wine intake. In fact, of all the different foods and drinks consumed by post-menopausal women, it was wine which had the strongest correlation with breast density. But the two wine types were different. Red wine drinkers tended to have less dense breasts, but it was the opposite for white wine drinkers. The density differences weren't huge, but the overall trend was significantly in red wine's favour. "The association with red wine is especially interesting, in the light of the favorable associations reported with red wine and other diseases", the researchers noted.*

That 1998 Mayo Clinic study was replicated a decade later by researchers at the equally prestigious Columbia University, New York.[4] While they found that drinkers in general had a modest (12%) increase in breast density, red wine drinkers' breasts were the reverse, with up to 10% decrease. "We observed a consistent inverse association for red wine intake and mammographic density," reported the researchers.

Another research group to support the French 'red wine prevents breast cancer' findings were doctors at the Cedars-Sinai Medical Centre in Los Angeles. In a small but well controlled "pilot study" in 2012 they reported finding that red wine has beneficial effects on some of the hormones known to be implicated in breast cancer.[5] "There are chemicals in red grape skin and seeds … that may decrease breast cancer risk," observed co-author Dr Glenn Braunstein.

---

* By the way, with younger pre-menopausal women, red wine's beneficial effects on breast density didn't show up.

Although these studies are preliminary, they do hint that red wine may have some very special breast-friendly properties.

Indeed, at least two studies on mice have shown that the natural ingredients of red wine can actually reduce breast cancer tumours.[6] [7]

However, as of 2013, the global evidence remains equivocal. Although four studies show either a beneficial or neutral effect of wine on breast cancer risk,[8] about the same number do not.

Bowel Cancer

Although drinking more than 50 grams of alcohol a day may raise the risk of this cancer, a large study in Denmark found "an anti-carcinogenic effect of wine", in that people who drink wine have effectively no risk.[9]

An almost as large Cambridge University study in Britain agrees, and indeed goes further, reporting that wine drinkers virtually halve their risk of the cancer[10] (covered more fully in Chapter 2).

Lymphoma

Originally called Non-Hodgkins Lymphoma, this refers to the 80 or so non-solid cancers – whose incidence is rising inexorably, by the way.* It's currently roughly the sixth most common cancer, affecting about 5% of the population – mainly the over-60s.

Very little work has been done on this disease, but it looks as though alcohol in general slightly increases the chances of dying from it, but that red wine decreases the risk. A 2010 study by Yale University found that the greatest reduction in risk (28%) occurred among people who had been drinking red wine for more than 25 years – preferably having started in their early twenties.[11]

However, that rather sophisticated investigation was done

---

* Possibly due to pesticide exposure.

only on women – and it's not been replicated. For example, two earlier Italian studies failed to find any benefit from wine, red or white.[12]

Lung cancer
Seventeen studies have looked at the connection between various types of alcohol intake and lung cancer. A 2007 summary of the data reported that red wine decreased the cancer risk by about 30%, with its protective effect strongest in older men and smokers.[13]

A later study on 84,170 American men confirmed the findings, showing found that for each glass of red wine consumed per month, the risk of lung cancer declined by 2%. The most substantial reduction in risk – a fairly impressive 60% – occurred in smokers drinking up to about a third of a bottle of red wine a day.[14]

Stomach Cancer
From 1964 to 1992, Danish researchers tracked the drinking habits of nearly 30,000 people to check their stomach cancer rates, and found that wine was hugely protective – and the higher the intake, the more the prevention: 75 grams a week resulted in a 24% reduction in risk, but drinking more than twice that produced a staggering 84% reduction in risk.[15]

Prostate Cancer
In 2005, a study of red wine intake and risk of prostate cancer among 1500 Americans reported finding that:

> each additional glass of red wine consumed per week showed a statistically significant 6% decrease in relative risk of prostate cancer, with evidence for a decline in risk estimates across increasing categories of red wine intake.[16]

In a press release accompanying the study, lead author Dr Janet Stanford said that the risk of prostate cancer was halved by drinking a mere four glasses (or more) of red wine a week – and particularly in the worst cases of the disease. "The more clinically aggressive prostate cancer is where the strongest reduction in risk was observed, [with a] 60% reduction in risk.", she said.

Similar findings have been reported by the Dutch government's "Netherlands Cohort Study". This tracked the health of almost 60,000 men for over six years, and found a significant but modest reduction in prostate cancer risk of about 17% among men who drank more than a couple of glasses of red wine a day.[17]

However, not all studies agree, so it's still a bit of a hung parliament on prostate cancer and red wine. Nevertheless, constituents of red wine have been found to help prevent prostate cancer in mice specially bred to get human prostate cancer,[18] which suggests there may be some Good News ahead.

Oesophageal cancer

While alcohol in general is Bad News for cancer in the throat and gullet area, wine drinking vastly reduces the risk, and may even be completely innocent, according to a 13 year study on 30,000 Danes.[19]

> A moderate intake of wine probably does not increase the risk of upper digestive tract (*gullet*) cancer, whereas a moderate intake of beer or spirits increases the risk considerably

reported chief scientist Professor Morten Grønbæk in 1998 – a finding fully confirmed a decade later by Spanish researchers.[20]

Wine's apparent protective effect makes sense because the risk of a condition called Barrett's Esophagus, a common precursor of the cancer, has been found to be halved by drinking a glass or more of wine a day – over 13 grams of alcohol.[21]

Dementia

Scandinavian scientists were among the first to investigate the red wine/dementia evidence. Sweden is well known for its exceptional "socialised" medical health care, and it has research funds to match. In 1968, the University of Gothenburg began a remarkable investigation into women's lifestyle and disease. Called the Population Study of Women, it tracked the health of a group of 1500 women aged between 38 and 60 … until they died.[22]

By 2002, about 10% of the women had developed dementia – enough to reveal any possible effects from alcohol. The results were clear-cut, showing a "robust protective association" among wine drinkers – as much as 70% reduction in risk. Spirits and beer drinkers didn't fare quite so well, however.

Danish researchers came up with much the same findings in a study of about 1600 over-65s, where a wine intake of up to about 20 grams a day roughly halved their risk of dementia.[23]

Predictably, the French have also investigated their national drink, which custom demands should accompany most main meals. So it's no surprise that this habit persists into old age, with the result that French OAPs often get through a good two-thirds of a bot a day. Far from tut-tutting, as the British medical establishment might do, French scientists from INSERM doubtless encourage their old folks with: "Bravo, allez-y, mes vieux!". That's because top-eurodollar research has shown that French geriatrics who drink between a quarter and half a litre of wine a day reduce their risk of dementia by a whopping 80%. Incidentally, half a litre of wine a day, although considered OTT in Britain, is deemed "moderate" in France, as the author of the dementia study, Professor Luc Letenneur makes clear in his conclusion that wine must be the key factor in preventing dementia. He says firmly:[24]

> The inverse relationship between moderate wine drinking
> and incident dementia [is] explained neither by known

predictors of dementia nor by medical, psychological or
socio-familial factors,

There's one big caveat, however, about dementia and red
wine: you've got to have the right genes.

This was discovered by researchers at New York's Columbia
University in 2004.[25] They studied about 1000 residents of
geriatric care homes in the city, in order to see if alcohol might
prevent dementia. Sure enough, like their French, Dutch and
Swedish counterparts, the American researchers confirmed
wine's special value in preventing dementia. However, there
were a few old people for whom wine didn't work: those
carrying a genetic variant called the APOE-epsilon 4 allele.
People carrying this gene are known to have an increased risk
of Alzheimers Disease – up to11 times the risk.[26] Sadly, wine
can't help these people, the gene's malign influence evidently
overpowering any protective benefits wine can muster.

Macular Degeneration

This progressive disease of the retina often afflicts people
as they get older, and can result in actual blindness. No-
one knows why MD occurs nor how to prevent it. Towards
the end of the last century, University of Washington DC
ophthalmologists decided to cast a beady eye over the
drinking habits of their patients, fully expecting to find
that the demon drink would be a major risk factor, but
"surprisingly" found the opposite:[27]

> Moderate wine consumption is associated with decreased
> odds of developing age-related macular degeneration.
> This is an important addition to the current scientific
> knowledge about MD.

Sexual function

Women first. The only people interested in probing wine's
effects on female sexual response appear to be Italians.
"Historically, the aspects of wine and sexuality have been
well known since the time of Ancient Greece, but the field
of female sexual dysfunction is still highly unexplored",

Dr. Nicola Mondaini and her colleagues at the University of Florence tell us.[28] In a study in 2009, they asked 800 women aged between 18 and 50 to answer a standard questionnaire which scores Female Sexual Function.[29] They excluded anyone who either smoked or drank excessively, concentrating on women who drank either a glass or two of red wine a day, or water.

What did they discover?

From a predatory male perspective, Mondaini's findings were in the right direction, albeit not terribly excitingly: teetotallers scored 68% on sexual satisfaction, single glass drinkers 72%, and double glassers 76%.

But once again, we come up against the issue of causality. Does red wine marginally improve a woman's sex life, or do the kind of women who choose to drink red wine also have a good sex life?

"A thorough comprehension of the mechanisms underlying female sexuality remains difficult," the study concludes – somewhat unnecessarily, one might think.

Male wine-drinkers haven't had their sex lives investigated by Dottore Mondaini – or by anyone else. The only data I can find is that a constituent of red wine increases the effectiveness of the erectile dysfunction drug, Levitra … but only if you're a rat.[30]

Heart Disease

This is the health area most often linked to red wine – not just in the scientific press, but the popular one too. Because the French are the world's biggest red wine consumers, that fact has been touted as an explanation for the so-called French Paradox.[31] [32] This concept first emerged in the 1990s as a response to Anglo-Saxon nutritionists who were mystified by the fact that the French weren't dropping dead like *mouches* from their high-fat diets. The proposed explanation was that red wine's healthy ingredients must be counteracting the "unhealthy" fats.

However, as we saw in chapter 3, the survey evidence is that heart disease appears to be prevented by alcohol itself, rather than by individual types.

But that's now been called into question by doctors at the University of Barcelona's Institut d'Investigacions Biomèdiques who embarked on a major alcohol research programme in the early part of this century. They decided to treat red wine like a new pharmaceutical experimental drug, and test its effects on human guinea-pigs in laboratory conditions. The researchers used a "placebo-controlled crossover experimental design" – a bog standard method for comparing the efficacy of two rival drugs. The Spanish comparison "drug" to wine was gin.

They did a whole series of clinical trials, whose overall upshot was to demonstrate that red wine has some tangible heart disease benefits over and above those of gin. i.e over alcohol itself. Here's a run-down of their main findings.

Red wine:

1. Reduces "inflammatory biomarkers of atherosclerosis"; in other words, it helps stop the body producing some of the substances that cause furred-up arteries. Gin is pretty good too, says the Spanish evidence, but red wine is even better.[33]

2. Improves "glucose metabolism and the lipid profile, conferring protective effects on cardiovascular disease". Both gin and red wine increase HDL ("good" cholesterol) and healthy lipoproteins, but only red wine decreases insulin levels – an extra plus for heart disease and diabetes prevention.[34]

3. "Decreases erythrocyte superoxide dismutase (SOD) activity". SOD is bad news for heart disease as it increases blood oxidation, creating harmful blood contents such as LDL ("bad" cholesterol). Red wine significantly counteracts this effect, thus making it a useful antioxidant. Gin is OK too, but it's not nearly as good.[35]

How much wine (and gin) produced these startling effects? 30 grams of alcohol a day – described by the Spanish medics as a "moderate" intake, but again right at the top of the UK authorities' safety limit for men.

Spanish women were also tested – although they received less booze than the men (20 grams of alcohol a day). Their human guinea-pig role was to see if white as well as red wine might benefit heart disease's "inflammatory biomarkers". The results clearly showed that both white and red wine have significantly beneficial effects on many of these heart disease precursors, but that red is more powerful.[36]

So the Barcelona data show unequivocal evidence that both alcohol itself and red wine in particular decrease the substances in blood which cause heart disease. This is an immensely important finding, because clinical trials such as the ones used by the Spanish researchers are the pinnacle of evidence-based medicine – you can't get any better proof than that.

For the first time, therefore, we have strong evidence of alcohol's direct benefits on the human body. This means we can now be much more confident about the epidemiological data. Indeed, an increasing number of medical authorities are convinced that the connection between alcohol and good health is no longer a mere "association", it is almost certainly causal. Alcohol is now thought to have "biologically plausible" health benefits – at least as far as heart disease is concerned, say Italian and American experts.[37] [38]

Indeed, on the Barcelona data alone, alcohol would seem to be much better at preventing heart disease than any prescription medication.

In fact, French scientists have already confirmed precisely that – on red wine drinkers. In a 20 year study on over 35,000 men with medium to high blood pressure (but taking no medication for it), the researchers found that wine drinkers "had significantly lower risks of death from all causes by [up to] 37%, than did abstainers."[39] How much *vin rouge* did the Frenchmen drink to get this remarkable effect? Nearly a bottle of wine (60 grams of alcohol) a day. Above that intake, the benefit tailed off.

One way red wine may do its work is by reducing levels of homocysteine, a known risk factor for heart disease. A 2002 study[40] found red wine reduced homocysteine levels by about 20%, and white wine slightly less. Another study discovered that alcohol in general and wine in particular increases blood levels of omega-3 fatty acids – well-established preventers of heart disease.[41] This is a really important finding, because Omega-3 fatty acids are rare in Western diets, being found mainly in oily fish. So the evidence suggests that alcohol is another source of this vital nutrient.

Kidney stones

As we saw in Chapter Five, alcohol in general helps prevent kidney stones, but wine is best, according to a Harvard study on over 45,000 men – beating beer and spirits by a fair margin.[42] Female wine drinkers fare even better, with an impressive 60% reduction in risk, say the same Harvard team.[43]

Weight Loss

Wine is the best alcohol for losing – or at least not gaining – weight, according to the few surveys that have compared alcohol types. For example, a 7 year study in 2012 on 15,000 middle-aged North American women, while confirming that alcohol in general helps reduce weight, found that "wine consumption showed the greatest protective association for the risk of [becoming] overweight" – a 25% reduction in risk. [44]

Similar results were found in other studies already covered in Chapter 7.

The Common Cold

This relatively harmless bi-, tri- or even quadri-annual affliction has a disproportionately large misery index, which is why drug companies have spent gazillions trying to find a cure … and failed. However, the answer had been staring them in the face all along – in their corporate hospitality room's wine rack. For yes indeed, wine does help prevent the common cold – and very substantially, according to a joint research venture between Harvard and Spanish universities in 2002.[45] The study recruited enough cold sufferers to enable the researchers to measure the health differences between red and white wine drinkers, and smokers and non-smokers. The results were astounding. Intake of both types of wine considerably reduced the chances of catching a cold. By and large the more wine drunk, the bigger the preventive effect – up to a 60% reduction risk of catching a cold among red wine drinkers, and a staggering 88% reduction in non-smoking white wine drinkers.

This astonishing finding was reinforced by an earlier placebo-controlled clinical trial in Britain's (now defunct) Common Cold Unit in 1993.[46] The researchers invited about 400 regular drinkers plus a smattering of teetotallers to come into their laboratory, deliberately infected them with a cold virus, and sat back to watch what happened. Utterly remarkable, it was the teetotallers who were most susceptible to getting a cold, and the heaviest drinkers the least. There was an absolutely straight line correlation between the amount of alcohol intake and protection against succumbing to the virus. And the effect was huge: people who drank 20 grams of alcohol a day had almost ten times fewer cold symptoms than teetotallers.

There is no drug, herb or medical intervention that can come close to offering that level of protection against mankind's commonest viral disease.

Longevity

Given all the above, it won't surprise you to learn that there's a good deal of evidence that red wine helps you live longer.

The first and most dramatic verification came in the year 2000 from researchers at the University of Copenhagen, led by Denmark's top alcohol expert, Professor Morten Grønbæk. This was a seriously in-depth study which pooled the data from three long-term surveys: 24,500 people aged between 20 and 98 were followed, and the cause and date of death was noted, plus how much and what type of alcohol they drank.[47]

The results were stunning.

First, they confirmed the medically incorrect fact that drinkers live longer than non-drinkers (as shown in Chapter 9). But second, wine drinkers live even longer still.

Here's the "abstract" (medic-speak for summary) of that study in full:*

---

*   This is the last one – promise!

During 257,859 person-years of follow-up, 4833 participants died. J-shaped relations were found between total alcohol intake and mortality at various levels of wine intake. Compared with non-drinkers, light drinkers who avoided wine had a relative risk for death from all causes of 0.90 (95% CI, 0.82 to 0.99) and those who drank wine had a relative risk of 0.66 (CI, 0.55 to 0.77). Heavy drinkers who avoided wine were at higher risk for death from all causes than were heavy drinkers who included wine in their alcohol intake. Wine drinkers had significantly lower mortality from both coronary heart disease and cancer than did non-wine drinkers ($P = 0.007$ and $P = 0.004$, respectively). Conclusion: Wine intake may have a beneficial effect on all-cause mortality that is additive to that of alcohol. This effect may be attributable to a reduction in death from both coronary heart disease and cancer."

Forgive me for burdening you with all this medical jargon, but the results are so extraordinary that I felt obliged to reprint the entire summary, so that sceptical medic readers can be in no doubt about the results (they'll find the p numbers impressive, by the way).

Here is a more graphic way of showing the data, taken from the same Copenhagen University study.

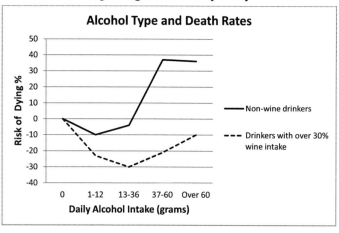

Adapted from Grønbæk M. et al. Type of Alcohol Consumed and

Mortality from All Causes, Coronary Heart Disease, and Cancer, *Annals of Internal Medicine,* September 19, 2000 vol. 133 no. 6 411–419.

This is a graph of drinkers' risk of dying, broken down into drinkers who never drank wine, and drinkers for whom wine was at least roughly a third of their total alcohol intake. Both lines are plotted against teetotallers' death rates (the zero line in this graph)

Look at the chart of the non-wine drinkers. Once again, as we saw in Chapter 9, there is the characteristic J-curve of alcohol intake reducing death risk compared to teetotallers, but only up to a point: in this case an intake of about 35 grams of alcohol a day. Above that, there's an increase in risk of death compared to non-drinkers.

By contrast, the people who included wine in their alcohol intake had a U-shaped curve of death risk. First, an even lower risk of dying, maximising at an intake of about 35 grams of alcohol per day. Second, and most dramatically, their death risk never exceeded that of non-drinkers, even at the very highest alcohol intakes.

Astonishing results which make one think: where's the mistake? Well, a very similar pattern of results has been found by medical researchers in California.

In 2003, Dr. Arthur Klatsky and colleagues at Oakland's Kaiser Permanente Medical Center reported the results of a 20-year long study on 128,000 people, during which over 16,000 of them died.[48] Correlating deaths with people's alcohol intake, Klatsky's data shows (when you take out deaths from "unnatural causes") a slight reduction in death risk among drinkers of any type of alcohol up to 42 grams a day, and a slight increase above 84 grams a day. But looking at wine drinkers only, Klatsky reported:

> Independent of total alcohol intake, wine drinking frequency was associated with lower risk of total mortality and several other endpoints, most notably coronary disease and respiratory deaths ... [with] a slightly lower risk of cancer ... Perhaps most convincing was the lower

> risk associated with wine drinking frequency at each of three total drinking levels (less than one, one or two, and three or more drinks *[over 42 grams]* per day).

Klatsky's results were not as dramatic as Grønbaek's in Denmark, in that he was unable to confirm whether there is no upper limit to wine intake and longevity – for the entirely practical reason that "only two deaths occurred in heavy, exclusive wine drinkers, [thus] limiting data interpretation".

Both studies should be bombshells to the medical establishment's position on alcohol and health, so why haven't we heard of them? One of the excuses could be the "confounding" issue.

This is how Grønbaek's publishers interpreted his results in a statement prepared for the lay public:

> It is possible that it is not wine drinking itself but some other characteristic of people who drink wine (for example, the types of food they eat or their income levels) that allows them to live longer than people who don't drink wine.[49]

Similarly, Klatsky echoed:

> Persons in Northern California who drink preponderantly wine are more often women, college graduates, non-smokers, and temperate drinkers, characteristics even more pronounced in persons drinking wine exclusively. In Denmark, wine drinking is associated with better perceptions of overall health, higher socio-economic status and intelligence quotients, and intake of a "healthy" diet (high in fruits, vegetables, fish, salads, and olive oil). Higher socio-economic status is associated with good health, and healthy habits tend to be clustered in the same person.

So, the argument goes, it's possible that the apparent longevity benefits from wine are an artefact created by the fact that wine drinkers are affluent and intelligent, have healthy lifestyles, tend not to binge drink etc etc.

On the other hand, this objection is so blindingly obvious

that do you imagine Klatsky and Grønbaek didn't know about it? Of course they did. Indeed they designed their research protocols specifically to try and take account of it, and devote whole chunks of their papers to discussing the thorny issue. "Estimates were adjusted for age, sex, educational level, smoking status, physical activity, and body mass index," writes Grønbaek, "(but) there may be an unrecognised lifestyle factor strongly related to mortality, other than those already controlled for." Klatsky claims to have factored in every conceivable confounder, but had to admit there may be some unknown "residual confounding." However, he's pretty sure his data is artefact-free, ending his paper with this robust conclusion:

> The unexpected strength and consistency in our data [connecting wine and longevity] … raises the likelihood of a causal association.

So, let's go along with Professor Klatsky, take the longevity data at face value, and assume that the Even Better News about wine is a genuine finding. The obvious question is this: what's special about wine?

What's in Wine?

Everyone agrees wine's a bit of a puzzle. It's been described as a "nutritionally complex food".[50] Most of wine's constituents are water and alcohol, of course, but the liquid contains a huge array of natural chemicals derived from grapes.

Professor Maynard Amerine, the late Professor of Oenology and Viticulture at the University of California at Davis (the USA's top wine research centre), said:

> Wine is a chemical symphony composed of ethyl alcohol, several other alcohols, sugar, other carbohydrates, polyphenols, aldehydes, ketones and pigments, with half a dozen vitamins, fifteen to twenty minerals, more than twenty-two organic acids, and other things that have not yet been identified.[51]

That was in 1986, since when the wine picture has got a bit less cloudy.

Here are the vitamins and minerals in wine:

Thiamine	Riboflavin	Niacin
Choline	Magnesium	Potassium
Calcium Chloride	Silicic Acid	Fluoride
Aluminum	Manganese	Sodium
Iron	Boron	Iodine
Copper	Rubidium	Betaine

Of course, these nutrients are in very small amounts, but they're still at useful health levels – the minerals in particular.

But it's not those constituents that have got nutritionists excited, it's these:

Polyphenols in Wine
Milligrams per litre

Compound	Red Wine	White Wine
Nonflavonoids	240–500	160–260
Hydroxybenzoic acids	0–260	0–100
p-Hydroxybenzoic acid	20	–
Gallic acid	116	1.4
Total gallates	40	7
Salicylic acid	–	–
Syningic acid	5	–
Protocatechuric acid	88	–
Hyproxycinnamic acids	162	130–154
cls/trans-Coutaric	20	1.8
cls/trans-Caftaric	25	5
Caffeic acid	8.5	2.8
Coumaric acid	12.6	1.5
Ferulic acid	19	–
Stilbenes	12.3	1.8

Compound	Red Wine	White Wine
trans-Resveratrol	1.0	0.22
Flavonoids	750–1060	25–30
Flavonols	98	trace
Quercetin	18.8	0
Myricetin	16.2	0
Kamempferol	18	0
Rutin	6.8	0
Flavanols	168	15–30
Catechin	89	17.3
Epicatechin	57.3	13.6

I make no apology for peppering your pages with such recondite chemical names – they at least serve to demonstrate wine's multifarious contents. But why are they so interesting to nutritionists?

Because these natural chemicals within wine are all classified as polyphenols – compounds thought to be rather Good News for health.

Polyphenols are substances naturally produced by plants in order to protect themselves from stressors such as disease and the ultraviolet rays in sunshine. By the end of the last century, science had begun to discover that polyphenols are valuable health-promoting "antioxidants" – not just for plants but humans too.

An explanatory diversion. What's wrong with "oxidants" that they need "antis"?

Well, the culprit is believed to be a group of chemicals called free radicals. These sound like wayward political renegades, and in a sense biologically they are, because they're dangerous loose cannons. Free radicals are created mainly as a by-product of oxygen powering the bodily systems, and, unless neutralised, can go around chemically attaching themselves to molecules and oxidising them. For example, they're thought to oxidise cholesterol, creating LDLs (the 'bad' cholesterol). There's even a theory that free radicals are responsible for the ageing process itself.

So the body's free radicals need clobbering. But how? The principal weapons are antioxidants, which we derive from eating plants. Originally, it was thought that fruits, vegetables and cereals were the only source of antioxidants, but as the evidence has built up about wine's health benefits, nutritionists now think we have a hitherto unsuspected extra supply of antioxidant goodies – the polyphenols in wine.

And it turns out that wine has some of the best antioxidants around.

In 1999, British researchers at Guy's Hospital Medical School in London compared the antioxidant properties of wine against standard fruits and vegetables ... with remarkable results. They reported finding that:

> The antioxidant activities of 1 glass (150 ml) of red wine are equivalent to 4 apples, 5 portions of onion, 5.5 portions of aubergine, and 3.5 glasses of blackcurrant juice.[52]

They also found a stark difference between red and white wine, with red containing "12 times" more antioxidant polyphenols than white.

US nutritional biochemists Professors J. Bruce German and Rosemary Walzem agree :

> Wine is a rich source of a large number of individual polyphenols. In this regard, wine differs from other foods such as onions, that contain predominantly a single flavonoid. This simple fact of wine biology makes many of the fundamental interpretations about the health effects of wine complex.[53]

But science doesn't much care for complexity, often preferring to reduce phenomena down to their simplest components before investigating them.* So nutritionists have

---

* Hence the term "reductionist" to describe modern science. Once hailed as the pinnacle of research methodology, reductionism is increasingly becoming a dirty word, as critics argue it offers an incomplete

scrutinised wine's polyphenols, and chosen just one that might explain the apparently greater health benefits of red over white. The polyphenol that stood out was a compound called resveratrol – possibly because red wine contains quite a lot of it, and white wine far less.

Why the difference? Because there's a lot of resveratrol in grape skins and very little in the juice. While white wine is made mainly made from juice, red includes both the skin and the juice.

So resveratrol it was.

The first resveratrol study was done in 1978 – the only one that year. Since then, the rise in the yearly number of research studies has been exponential: 113 in 2000, 337 in 2007, and 726 in 2012 – a veritable academic tsunami. By the time this book went to press, reductionist science had notched up a staggering 5872 studies on resveratrol.[54]

You (and I) will be thankful that this book merely distils the findings. But they're damn interesting.

Resveratrol research
There's a kind of pecking order protocol in biology for exploring any new substance. It must first to be tested on body cells in test-tubes, then in animals, and finally in humans.

By 2013, resveratrol had reached the animal stage, and had just begun to get round to humans.

Here's an extract from a 2012 paper summarising the research findings:

> In experimental studies, resveratrol exhibits both cardio-protective and chemopreventive effects.... It inhibits the growth of some tumor types, and exhibits anti-inflammatory, antibacterial, antifungal, antiviral, neuroprotective, anti-proliferative and anti-angiogenic activities.[55]

In plain language: in laboratory tests, resveratrol has shown it can protect brain cells, combat most kinds of infections,

---

understanding of natural phenomena.

help to stop the development and spread of cancer, and prevent heart problems.

Remarkable.

It's yet more evidence reinforcing red wine's role in preventing heart disease. But cancer? That's really interesting. What exactly might resveratrol do to combat the big C?

Quite a lot, it turns out.

For example, in 1997, a group of scientists at the University of Illinois discovered that resveratrol has "cancer chemopreventive activity in assays representing three major stages of carcinogenesis", recommending that it "merits investigation as a potential cancer chemopreventive agent in humans."[56]

Most work has been done on breast cancer, where resveratrol has been found to "prevent the first step that occurs when estrogen starts the process that leads to cancer", reported Dr Eleanor Rogan at the University of Nebraska after her experiments testing the compound on breast cancer cells. According to Rogan, resveratrol works by inducing an enzyme called quinone reductase which inactivates estrogen, high levels of which are thought to be a risk factor for breast cancer. "This is dramatic because it was achieved with fairly low concentrations of resveratrol *(about what's in a glass of red wine)*" she writes.[57]

Another astonishing piece of breast cancer Good News is that other red wine polyphenols apart from resveratrol are remarkably similar to the latest breast cancer drugs: the so-called Aromatase Inhibitors. The drug industry has spent billons developing AIs, because they have the effect of reducing estrogen, a female hormone linked to breast cancer.

But Big Pharma may not have needed to bother, because AIs are already present in plentiful quantities within grapes – in the skins, the seeds and the juice.[58] [59]

Hardly surprising therefore that it's been found that red wine "completely abrogates neoplastic changes in [mice] mammary tissue" i.e. totally prevents mice breast cells developing cancer. That's a discovery by a group of scientists at

California's Beckman Institute, who went on to make the remarkable suggestion that:

> Red wine or red wine extract may be a chemo-preventive diet supplement for postmenopausal women who have a high risk of breast cancer.[60]

So, two groups of researchers have concluded that red wine constituents might help prevent breast cancer. Although by 2013 the red wine/ polyphenols research so far only applies to mice, it does confirm that Keats' "blushful Hippocrene" – or even plonk – are not necessarily Bad News for breast cancer, and might well be Good. The whole breast cancer issue will be revisited in Appendix One.

Reservations about resveratrol
There's been a fair degree of scepticism about resveratrol, however. The fact is that drug companies have chucked quite a lot of money at researching the compound, but have decided it's not particularly promising. What's more (and perhaps not unrelatedly), one prominent resveratrol research scientist has been found to have fiddled his data.* Finally, and most damningly, resveratrol is suspected of not being "bioavailable"– in other words, it's thought to be poorly absorbed by the body.[61]

However, two separate research groups don't think there is a bioavailability problem, having discovered that resveratrol has some very special modes of action – to the body's benefit. For example, one of the health problems associated with being carnivorous is that the very process of digesting red meat inevitably creates oxidising by-products which can be mildly carcinogenic.[62] Remarkably, in 2008, scientists at the Hebrew of University in Jerusalem found that when people drink quite modest amounts of red wine along with meat, those toxic by-products are significantly reduced.[63]

"These findings explain the important benefit of

---

* He's neither mentioned nor referenced in this book.

consuming dietary polyphenols during meals", say the Israeli researchers, having discovered that wine components such as resveratrol don't need to be conventionally "bioavailable" (i.e. reach the bloodstream) before they can be of health value.

Strong supporting evidence has come from Professor Karen Brown and her team at the University of Leicester who made the astounding discovery that resveratrol does a magic trick in the body, by recombining after it's metabolised.[64] Says Brown:

> A problem that is often stated for resveratrol is its poor bioavailability. It gets absorbed pretty well into the blood, but once there it is metabolised very quickly, so you get low levels of resveratrol in the blood, but you also get high levels of resveratrol's metabolites, called sulphates. We've shown that when these sulphates enter cells, the cells actually reprocess the sulphates back into resveratrol. We were surprised to find that this regenerated resveratrol is almost as bioactive as the original substance. Indeed, it's at high enough concentrations to stop cancer cells growing in our laboratory test-tubes.[65]

Brown's breakthrough discovery shows that, although tech-nically resveratrol is not bioavailable, its unique recombination trick means it still finds a way of delivering its Good News benefits. Pretty canny.

The final sceptical blast against resveratrol is that there's not nearly enough of it in red wine for it to be of any practical health value. Here are two typical comments: "You'd need to drink between 50 and 200 glasses of wine to get the same relative amount of resveratrol used by researchers",[66] and "At least 100 glasses would be needed each day to get the levels shown to improve health in mice".[67] These views are not supported by the evidence, however. For example, clinical trials have demonstrated that a dose of 16 milligrams a day can have significant health benefits for heart disease patients.[68] What's 16 milligrams of resveratrol? The average amount in a small glass of red wine.

In any case, the focus on resveratrol having been largely driven by drug company money (which has begun to dry up), the more forward-thinking researchers have been broadening their horizons … away from reductionist science, towards a realisation that, as far as wine and health are concerned, other constituents than resveratrol are important – not least because they may all work synergistically.

For example, red wine's benefits on weight have been found to be related to a substance called piceatannol, a metabolite of resveratrol, which "blocks an immature fat cell's ability to develop and grow", according to Purdue University scientists.[69]

Similarly, red wine's phenomenal success in preventing the common cold has been ascribed to its "rich content" of flavonoid polyphenols such as quercetin and catechin; these have powerful anti-viral effects, because they can penetrate virus molecules, "interfering with the synthesis of viral nucleic acid".[70]

World expert Professor Ramon Estruch and his colleagues at the University of Barcelona have this to say about the burgeoning research data about wine:

> The beneficial effects of moderate wine consumption may be attributed to the overall mix of all of its components and not to a specification of one, such as resveratrol. Indeed, progress can be achieved in the health effects of polyphenols when the one-dimensional antioxidant view of polyphenols is replaced by a view considering their multifaceted bioactivity, as polyphenols are versatile bioactives rather than mere antioxidants. Furthermore, rather than polyphenols themselves, their metabolites might be the real key players in cardiovascular and cancer protection.[71]

A sentiment echoed by Dr Gerald Weissmann, editor-in-chief of the *FASEB Journal,* in 2010.

> When it comes to finding treatments for complex diseases, the answers are sometimes right there waiting to be discovered in unexpected places ... like the wine racks of the nearest store. The profound impact that the antioxidants in red wine have on our bodies is more than anyone would have dreamt just 25 years ago. As long as [it is] taken in moderation, all signs show that red wine may be ranked among the most potent 'health foods' we know.[72]

"Polyphenols are medicine; is it time to prescribe red wine for our patients?" ask Professors Alfredo Cordova and Bauer Sumpio, cardiologists at America's prestigious Yale University, answering their own question by recommending their fellow doctors to:

> encourage regular and moderate consumption of red wine, perhaps one or two drinks a day with meals.[73]

Having fought your way through this huge, very dense chapter, you may well think you deserve those two drinks right now!

13

Even Better News about Beer

Glance at this:

Micronutrients
Folate
B6
Niacin
Pantothenic acid
Riboflavin
Vitamin B12
Potassium
Magnesium
Phosphorus
Selenium
Silicon

Polyphenols
(+) Catechin
Ferulic acid
Vanillic acid
Isoxanthohumol
p-Coumaric acid

Syringic acid
Gallic acid
Sinapic acid
Protocatecuic acid
(-)-Epicatechin
6-Prenylnaringenin
Xanthohumol
4-Vinylguaiacol
Caffeic acid
8-Prenylnaringenin
Vinil-4-fenol
Vinil-4-guayacol
Etil-4-fenol
Isoeugenol
Tyrosol
Propil-4-siringol
2,3-Dihydroxy-guaiacyl1
propan-1-one
4-Hydroxyfenilacetic
Homovanillic
3-Metilcatecol
4-Etilcatecol
4-Metilcatecol
Vinil-4-fenol
3,5-Dihydroxybenzoic
2,6-Dihydroxybenzoic
2-Hydroxybonzoic
3-Hydroxybenzoic
4-Hydroxybenzoic
Gallic
Siningico
4-Hydroxybenzoic acid

0-Vanillin
Siringic aldehyde
m-Coumaric
o-Coumaric
5-Caffeoilquinic
Isoxanthohumol
8-Prenilnaringenin
6-Prenilnaringenin
6-Geranilnaringenin
T\xifolin
 (-)-Epicatechin
Catechin gallate
Epicatechin gallate
Procyanidin B3
Prodelphynidina B3
Prodelphnynidina B9
Procynadin C2
Kanpherol
Kanpherol-3-rhamnoside
Quercetin]3,7-
Dimetilquercetin
Miricetin
Quercetin 3-0-Arabinoside
Quercetina 3-0-Rutinoside
Quercitrin
Isoquercitrin
Rutin
Daidzein
Genistein
Formononetin
Biochanin A
Apigenin
a-acids (humulones)
Iso-a-acids (iso-humulones)
Catechol
Pirogalol

They're some of the goodies in beer. A pretty impressive list, eh? And that's not all of beer's contents. In fact, more than 2000 compounds have been discovered in the golden liquid – twice the number in wine.

However, although the antioxidant content of beer may be greater than wine's, the specific antioxidants are different – simply because beer's raw materials (barley and hops) contain different polyphenols from grapes. And that may be the problem.

What problem? Well, sadly for lovers of the foaming liquid, it appears that beer has few extra health benefits over and above those of alcohol itself.

That's odd because as far as **heart disease** is concerned, beer may even have a slight edge over wine. A meta-analysis (pull-together of all the evidence) in 2011 showed that people who drink 43 grams of alcohol a day in the form of beer have a substantial 42% "maximal protection [against] vascular risk". [1] 43 grams is way above the maximum UK recommended intake for men, and more than double the female top whack.

Beer's benefit in heart disease is believed to be due to its relatively high concentrations of folate, a B vitamin which combats homocysteine, a now well-established precursor of cardiovascular disease.[2]

Beer also appears to be highly protective against **Barrett's Esophagus**, a precursor of oesophageal cancer. One study found "a significant linear trend with [lifetime] beer consumption", revealing two staggering figures: up to an 80% reduction in risk on intakes up to 82 grams a day.[3]

A research group at Queens University Belfast also discovered that beer is pretty good at preventing helicobacter pylori, the bacteria mainly responsible for **stomach ulcers** – but only at tiny intakes of 8 grams a day (less than half a pint), and no more. [4]

In addition, anyone worried about getting **Parkinson's Disease** could well benefit from drinking a few bevvies a day, according to the findings of a huge US study in 2013, which found that 28 grams of alcohol in beer a day can reduce the risk of PD by nearly 30%.[5]

But er … that seems to be it, as far as beer is concerned.

As I say, that's puzzling because beer contains a barrel-load of nutrients – far more than wine. I offer three explanations for it being apparently less health-giving than wine.

First, beer drinkers tend not to look after themselves too well – for example by having a poor diet. A Danish survey of 3.5 million supermarket transactions showed that beer "tended to be purchased with chips and soft drinks".[6] Second, alcohol researchers themselves might prefer the grape to the grain, and so have scant interest in studying beer's benefits. Or lastly, it could be that, as the radical 16th century German cleric Martin Luther observed: *Bier ist menschenwerk, wein aber ist von Gott.*

"Beer is made by man, but wine is from God."

14

Even Better News about Spirits

None ...[*]

[This page has been intentionally left blank:
please use it for notes or doodles]

---

[*] Why? Because spirits are just alcohol and water – durr! Although they may contain traces of polyphenols from their plant sources, these would be at minuscule levels.

15

Reflections On, In and With a Glass

Congratulations on getting this far in the book.

I am painfully aware that it's been perhaps over-stuffed with Too Much Information. But my duty has been to provide enough detail to offer a goodly grasp of the medical evidence about alcohol and health – for the sake of your own health. If you need any more information, or want to check up on what you've read, you should visit a website called PubMed. This extraordinary online medical library contains a staggering 22 million articles, all of which can be accessed for free. PubMed was handed as a gift to the world by the US Government in 1997, and it has truly democratised public knowledge about medicine, thus usurping doctors' hitherto monopolistic control of health information; it's a kind of State-sponsored medical Wikileaks.

So you're now a lot wiser about the demon drink and its overplayed perils and underplayed benefits. While writing this book, and coming across such a treasure trove of really Good News About Booze, the puzzle has been: why haven't doctors ever come clean about all this?

One fairly obvious reason is that they don't trust us. Doctor friends I've consulted believe that's the primary reason. First, they fear that spilling the beans about the Good News might encourage youngsters to drink even more, and become even more of a bloody nuisance on the streets. Next, they think that, if the rest of us are told a few daily snifters will prolong our lives, we might imagine a lot will make us live even longer.

There's a third, darker reason, though. "Don't you know

that many doctors are or were alcoholics?," medic chums whisper. "There's nothing like an ex-addict to moralise about his habit." Of course, one must add hastily for the sake of Messrs Sue Grabbit and Runne,* that must not be taken to apply to any of the individuals referred to directly or indirectly in this book, whose personal lives I haven't a clue about.

Nevertheless, here's a quote from the online *Daily Mail* in 2011: "The British Medical Association has estimated that one in 15 doctors will develop an [alcohol] addiction problem". Beneath it was this very revealing blog from a retired country doctor:

> I am no longer working as a doctor but when I did, I was plastered every night. Used to sink best part of half a bottle of voddie every single night. I used voddie because it tends not to smell as much as whisky the next day. Couldn't go to work in the morning without using mouthwash. Couldn't drive my car as I was over the limit, so had to ride my bike. I fell into the hedge quite a few times. But it's hard work being a doctor, pretty stressful, I'm surprised that ALL doctors aren't drunks personally.[1]

In fact, there's a charity called the Sick Doctors Trust which was established in 1996 specifically to help the many doctors who have a drink problem.

I rest my case.

It makes total sense, therefore, that the entire MD clan might have a visceral collective terror of falling into the abyss of alcohol dependency, and thus keep the rest of us in the dark about booze's benefits as a kind of proxy for their own dark demons.

The Media

---

* The witty soubriquet for libel lawyers coined by satire mag, *Private Eye*.

The other clan who have a drink problem are, of course, journalists. Admittedly, the days of liquid lunches at El Vinos are long gone, but the stresses of the job and the socialising it demands means that overdoing the drink is a still a major occupational hazard.

So it's not surprising that, every now and then, some anti-alcohol flotsam and jetsam rises to the surface.

Here's a small breast-beating selection from 2013.

Is your drinking out of control?", asked 49-year old 'former journalist', Gabrielle Glaser, confessing to *The Times* readers about her own "excessive drinking".[2] Judith Woods in *The Telegraph* berated "the ladies who have too good a lunch" and the "rare middle-class mother who doesn't reach for a tipple of something come 'wine o'clock', when the kids are in bed."[3]

The same newspaper devoted substantial column inches to a soul-baring *cri de coeur* from a certain Bryony Gordon. "How binge-drinking became a *(her)* way of life" she wailed.[4]

And so on ... ad nauseam.

Journalists therefore will be a soft touch for any Bad News about booze, playing into the hands of the prohibitionist medics.

As a result, we get stories such as the one mentioned in Chapter 4 about diabetes. It claimed, you may remember, that binge drinking causes diabetes – entirely on the basis of a few animal experiments and a massive confusion about the definition of 'binge'.

Chapter 2 gave a couple of examples of stories about alcohol and DNA, which omitted to mention that the body has two robust natural defence mechanisms against any DNA damage caused by alcohol. But a DNA myth was born ... subsequently fostered by people who ought to know better.

"There is strong scientific evidence that alcohol itself is a cancer risk factor – possibly through damaging our DNA – in cancers of the breast, bowel, mouth, pharynx, larynx, oesophagus and liver," trumpeted a WCRF Press Release in January 2013. As we've already seen, that statement is only partially supported by the evidence.

Of course, journalists have neither the time nor the background knowledge to question the vast majority of press releases about medicine. But, for Bad News stories about alcohol, neither do they have the motivation, because Bad News supports their professional guilt trip.

And it gets worse. Not only does the press blindly trot out anti-alcohol press releases, it sometimes reports them with firework displays. Here's one example from many.

In 2012 a young PhD student and her London University supervisor decided to make a bit of a splash about the fact that people under-report their alcohol intake, although this phenomenon has been well-known since the early 1980s. The pair got hold of a couple of 2008 'How much do you drink?' surveys on about 20,000 people, and applied the 1980s under-reporting formula to the interviewees' self-reported figures.[5] Lo and behold, they found that Britain's total alcohol intake was higher than British drinkers themselves claimed. What a surprise. The fact that their study results were wholly "putative" and "hypothetical" was totally lost in the resulting media brouhaha. These were some of the horror headlines:

> Booze-fuelled Britain: Now 80% of women are 'binge drinking'

> Are you in drink denial? Half of adults down too much alcohol yet barely a quarter admit doing so

> A nation of 'secret boozers': English people underestimate how much alcohol they drink

However, the real horror story here is not the implications for drinkers, but for the whole science underpinning alcohol research. This is a hugely important issue which we'll return to shortly.

The alcoholic alliance between doctors and journalists gets unholier still, partly because, of all the professions, medicine seems immune to journalism's perfectly proper default position of benign scepticism. While writing his book, I've naturally kept my ears and eyes open for media stories on the subject, and not one of the medical interviewees has had their opinions questioned by journalists, either directly or indirectly. Why is this such a problem? Because almost every alcohol "media expert" tends to be an anti-alcohol evangelist, so the full News about Booze – both Good and Bad – never gets a look-in … a situation this book has attempted to redress.

Where do we go from here?

Although I've attempted to keep my personal take on alcohol and health research out of the long litany of studies you've had to wade through, you'd be surprised if, after months as it were immersed in alcohol, I hadn't formed some opinions.

So, for what they're worth, and in a suitably humble spirit of constructive criticism, here are a few final observations.

I have been a science and medical journalist all my life, and had the rare privilege of meeting world experts in a wide range of sciences, and covering their research in some depth – from lasers to linguistics, nutrition to animal navigation, and space science to parapsychology [*That's quite enough silly alliteration and prattish self-promoting puffery, Ed.*] … and frankly I've not come across a branch of science or medicine that is in such a mess as alcohol research.

Here's a short-list of the most obvious disaster areas.

Alcohol quantities
The way these are described is a true Tower of Babel.

As explained in Chapter 1, the division of alcohol content into "units", "drinks" or "servings" is a dog's breakfast of differing amounts of alcohol depending on which country you live in. That's confusing enough for the general public, but it gets medical researchers themselves tied up in knots too. Quickly glance at this extract from an international study purporting to provide reliable information to fellow-medics about the effects of alcohol on health (and its glaring mistake):

> Where consumption was reported in drinks and not grams, the gram pure alcohol equivalent described in the article was used as a conversion factor if stated, and if not, conversion from standard drinks was based on geography: for Canada 13.6 grams, the UK 8 grams, the USA 12 grams (*wrong, it's 14 grams*) and in both New Zealand and Australia 10 grams of pure alcohol were assumed based on the literature. For all other countries without clear standard drink specifications 12 grams pure alcohol was used.[6]

It gets worse. The adjectives used to categorise drinkers and their intakes are a mess too. Terms like "modest", "moderate" and "heavy" are tossed around in serious medical journals with scant regard for scientific rigour. For example, "moderate" alcohol intake is classified as "less than 60 grams a day" in one study[7] but "30 grams a day" in another.[8] However, a third study categorises people who drink over 30 grams a day as "very heavy drinkers".[9]

Such huge discrepancies don't need much hunting down, I assure you: the research literature is positively riddled with them.

These inconsistencies might be acceptable in a work of fiction, but they're a scandal in science. Why? Two reasons. First, scientists bandy these terms amongst themselves as if they had objective meaning, and second, the jumble of terms makes it difficult for health authorities to provide sensible advice about drink intakes. No wonder the official UK guidelines haven't changed one iota since they were first "plucked out of the air" in 1987.

Even scientists themselves are exasperated.

> For many years the lack of consensus in defining the moderate consumption of alcohol has, in most of the cases, made it difficult to compare results in studies all over the world,

complain Spanish alcohol researchers (incidentally the

world's leading experimental scientists on alcohol). However, once again exposing the Tower of Babel, they continue:

> For example, in the UK, moderation is defined as 21 units of alcohol a week for men and 14 units a week for women, a unit being 10 g of alcohol *(it's 8 g)*. In the USA, the most recent dietary guidelines define moderate drinking as up to 2 drinks a day for men and 1 drink a day for women. The problem emerges because there is no definition of the alcohol content of a drink. [Also] the type of beverage is not taken into account when defining moderation.[10]

Amen to that last sentence, but yet another howler confirms how often the quality of medical discourse about alcohol is a joke.

Research on animals

If alcohol researchers really must do animal experiments,*at least afford the creatures the courtesy of not suppressing the findings they've sacrificed themselves for. A classic example is in the field of breast cancer. As we saw in chapter 2, normally reared animals have never been found to get breast cancer after drinking alcohol; indeed, one well conducted long-term experiment on mice genetically 'programmed' to get breast cancer showed that alcohol had not a smidgeon of an effect on their cancer rates.[11]

That study was done in 1992, since when it has been totally ignored. Despite the fact that many experts have expressed the opinion that animal experiments are crucial in making sense of the confused human alcohol/breast cancer findings, not one of the many subsequent scientific reviews of the data has ever mentioned the study. One reviewer whom I questioned about the omission excused himself on the grounds that he "was allowed only 50 references". Readers might find that somewhat unconvincing, especially

---

* An activity of questionable moral justification in such a non life-threatening area as alcohol, especially since any potential adverse impact on human health is entirely self-inflicted.

in view of the fact that the reviewer was seeking to establish a link between alcohol and breast cancer ... which of course that 1992 mouse study comprehensively demolishes.

The other issue with animal research is this. If the creatures fail to give you the results you think they ought to, don't do nasty things to them until they do. Alcohol/cancer research is particularly guilty of this. Animals are already different enough from human beings without adding another layer of artificiality. Poisoning or infecting them in order to get the 'medically correct' finding is bad science, as it won't tell you anything meaningful anyway; it's just a PR stunt to dish more dirt on alcohol.

Causality

As has been emphasised every so often in the book, most of the evidence for alcohol's effects on human health relies on nothing more than intelligent guesswork. No matter how many surveys of drinking patterns and ill-health ('epidemiology') you carry out, it's impossible to 100% prove that booze is the cause of any particular health problem – nor benefit for that matter, of course. The most that epidemiological studies can tell you is that there is an 'association' between a behaviour such as drinking and the health manifestation. They can never prove that the behaviour causes it. That's an incontrovertible principle of both science and logic.

However, some alcohol researchers – even quite eminent ones – appear to have forgotten this.

For example, in 2006 two groups of top-flight British academics published a meta-analysis of the entire breast cancer/alcohol research database to date. The abstract (i.e. summary) of the analysis ended with this statement: "We conclude that the association between alcohol and breast cancer may be causal". That would have been the message promulgated to the world's press and health authorities, of course.

But if you actually read the thousands of words in the whole study, the story looks somewhat different – in particular that the evidence for a causal link between alcohol and breast cancer was pretty sketchy. Here's the small print of the study's conclusion, with two key words in bold:

> Although the excess risk associated with drinking alcohol is relatively small compared with the major risk factors for breast cancer, it is one of the few modifiable risk factors associated with breast cancer. Given the high prevalence of drinking, even a small risk linking breast cancer with alcohol, **if causal,** has serious public health implications in terms of the number of breast cancer cases attributable to drinking alcohol.

We'll be revisiting breast cancer and causality in Appendix One, by the way. But for the moment, consider the mess at the heart of this paper. When scientists talk to each other, they use the language of science. For example, in this paper, the words "if causal" is code for 'we know epidemiology can't actually prove anything'. However, because only the abstract would be read by the press or the health authorities (and via them, the public), my guess is that the 'politically correct' spin was applied to the abstract, and the words "if causal" were allowed to morph into "may be causal". That doesn't sound much of a move linguistically, but medically it's a huge leap across the Rubicon.

There's more in that vein – but far worse. The 2007 WCRF Report cited many times in Chapter 2, and which claims to be one of the most "authoritative" assessments of the alcohol/cancer connection, leaps from mere association to "convincing" causal proof. One example is bowel cancer, where the causal claim is based on the results of published studies many of which don't even reach so-called statistical significance – which, in other words, are scientifically meaningless. This extraordinary non-science nonsense was revealed in WCRF's own subsequent 2010 "Update on Alcohol and Colon Cancer"[13] which tacitly admits that more than half the studies in the earlier Report weren't statistically significant.

We're arguably in pseudoscience territory here.

Indeed, if these non-significant papers had been about acupuncture, homeopathy or the like, they would have been ridiculed – and rightly so (although I suspect that editors of alternative medical journals would have rejected the studies in the first place!)

But in the drive to blacken booze, anything goes.

It's bad enough leaping from 'association' to 'causation' anyway; it's only legitimate when there's really strong circum-stantial or clinical evidence, such as with smoking and lung cancer, or wine and heart disease. To cross the epistemological Rubicon and pretend that the flimsy and often contradictory alcohol/cancer data is evidence for causation is yet another joke.

Under-reporting

Earlier in this chapter I referred to a hyped-up story about people in Britain being "in denial" about their drinking, based on a London University survey in 2012. Leaving aside the press hysteria, the more sober conclusion of the study was that people under-reporting their alcohol intake has "enormous implications for public health in England" – adverse imp-lications, we're meant to believe, of course.

Contrast that with the implications drawn by a 20-strong group of Cambridge University researchers two years earlier. Talking specifically about alcohol intake and the risk of cancer, their take on the under-reporting problem is that it is liable to result in an "overestimation of the actual carcinogenic effect [of alcohol]."[14]

Yes, you read that right. Under-reporting means that the alcohol/cancer data make booze appear to be more of a health hazard than it really is.

For example, if Joe Bloggs says he drinks a half a bottle of scotch a day and drops dead from throat cancer, the chances are that it was a whole bottle of scotch that killed him, not the half a bottle he told people he drank. But that half a bot will be the amount of booze used as an intake figure in throat cancer studies.

I know what you're thinking: scientists can't be so silly, surely … this guy must be exaggerating.

'Fraid not, sorry.

In 1982 alcohol expert Dr Lorraine Madanik (now Professor and Dean at UC Berkeley) did a huge pioneering study, checking countries' real alcohol consumption against the figures derived from questionnaire-type surveys.[15] What she found astounded her research colleagues, who until then had imagined that people reliably reported how much they drank. They could hardly have been more wrong. Madanik discovered that there was a veritable chasm between actual and self-reported intakes "ranging from 40–60%".

In other words, people were found in reality to drink about 50% more alcohol than they actually confessed to interviewers. That staggering figure was confirmed twenty years later by Professor Ronald Knibbe of Maastricht University who discovered that Germans tend to under-report by 39% and the French by 56%.[16]

Now commonsense would suggest that, if it's well-known that people lie/forget/are wildly inaccurate about their drinking habits, medical researchers would take that into account when assessing booze's health hazards – or at least do something to correct the problem.

Not a bit of it.

Despite the under-reporting phenomenon being well established in 1982, and subsequently reconfirmed in 2001, nobody changed tack. Although occasional papers drew attention to the alcohol figures' "potentially large imprecision"[17] and the fact that "studies of the accuracy of self-report measures using verification techniques are virtually non-existent in the alcohol research field",[18] year after year, study after study, alcohol health researchers have lumbered on … painstakingly recording people's statements about how much alcohol they drank, while knowing it was seriously flawed – and yet using the data as the basis of supposedly scientific research. *

---

* Of course, professional groups such as Doll's physicians or Harvard's nurses may not under-report as much as Joe Public, but that simply

Surely the credibility of any research must be seriously undermined when the principal 'variable' (in this case, alcohol consumption) is so unknown. Science can tolerate a certain amount of uncertainty, of course, but only within narrow limits – never as much as 50% adrift (even 75% has been reported)[19] in the primary data. Once again, we're arguably in pseudoscience territory.

This has some major implications for issues about alcohol and health – not least that the evidence base is a real mess … but let's try and salvage something from the wreckage.

If you amalgamate the Midanek and Knibbe findings, you arrive at a rough under-reporting figure of 50%. So, on the assumption that people consistently under-report their intake by that amount, let's try to tidy up the alcohol consumption figures accordingly. What does such tidying do to the conclusions about alcohol's effects on the body – both the Bad News and the Good News?

First effect: the Bad News turns into somewhat less Bad News. Take a simple example. Assuming it's true that every glass of booze raises your risk of breast cancer by 10%, tidying now says you can drink a glass and a half for the same risk.

Similarly, lifespan. Chapter 9 showed evidence that an intake of about 65 grams of alcohol a day for European men is no more injurious to health (as measured by death rates) than being teetotal. 65 grams a day is a self-reported figure, of course; so, applying our 50% tidying formula, the figure magically climbs to 97.5 grams. Therefore, using the reference charts on the inside covers of this book, mathematical logic brings one to the conclusion that European men might be able to drink nearly half a bottle of scotch, almost five pints of beer, or a litre of wine a day without damaging their health one bit. By the same token, European women might be able to drink 30 grams a day without the slightest risk of shortening their lives. These figures are way over any country's officially

---

amplifies the uncertainty of the database.

advised maximum intakes, of course.

On the Good News front, the implications are that we need to drink more (red wine in particular) in order to obtain the necessary health benefits. For example, if a daily intake of the 20 grams of alcohol in red wine helps prevent dementia,[20] the therapeutic dose must now be raised to 30 grams. Even more importantly for people's longevity (and so by definition everyone's general health), the lifespan graphs from Chapter 9 (page 109) must now be reworked. In order to live as long as possible, European men now need to drink between 5 and 30 grams a day, and women about half that amount.

Of course, the 50% tidying formula can't be accurate because there are way too many uncertainties within it. But, given the Midanek and Knibbe evidence, it's bound to be closer to a true alcohol intake figure than what's currently claimed by alcohol research.

Alcohol is not the only area of public health where the raw materials of research are so fundamentally flawed, of course. Food intake is another one, where under-reporting is also routine.[21] But tough, that's life.

What should alcohol research do about the problem? First, it should come clean about it. In all the many thousands of medical studies on alcohol, there is scarcely a mention of it. And of course, Joe Public never gets to hear of it.

Medicine should have the humility to admit the problem, and not pretend that its prognostications have the status of Absolute Truth. It's surely not legitimate to issue *ex cathedra* instructions about people's alcohol intakes when the supporting evidence base is so tawdry.

Begging the question

In Chapter 9, we saw how medical science has come up with the superficially scary concept of 'alcohol-related diseases'. Once again, these terms are bandied about as if they had the status of Absolute Truth. However, as you may remember, that chapter showed evidence of experts admitting (albeit whispering amongst themselves, of course) that only a "small minority" of drinkers actually get these conditions.

How can this possibly come about? Are doctors lying? No.

Let me suggest how diseases can become 'alcohol-related' without any deception whatever – just crummy logic and bad science.

Take the fictitious case of 65 year-old Fred Smith who dies of liver disease in hospital. The doctor has to sign the death certificate, of course. What does he (or she, sorry!) write on it? The doctor's logic circuits will go like this:

1. Mr Smith died of liver disease.
2. Did Mr Smith drink alcohol?
3. Yes (a racing certainty, as 75% of adult men drink)[22]
4. *Ergo*, Mr Smith died of Alcoholic Liver Disease.

Thus, in death, Mr Smith has given birth to yet another phoney alcohol statistic.

This is not just bad science, it's also bad for public policy, because you end up with 'official statistics' like the one we saw in Chapter 9 from a UK Government document called *Alcohol-related deaths in the United Kingdom, 2011:*

> Alcoholic Liver Disease is the most prevalent of all alcohol-related causes of death and is responsible for approximately 66% of all alcohol-related deaths in 2011.[23]

But that's an unlikely figure, given that "only a small proportion of alcoholic patients develop advanced liver disease, suggesting that factors other than alcohol intake may influence Alcoholic Liver Disease", as we saw in Chapter 9.[24]

The problem is that official statistics are the only ones put in front of politicians, and if they're wrong (intentionally or not), they lead policy-makers by the nose to the belief that alcohol is nothing but Bad News for health.

Which as we've seen, in the words of the song, ain't necessarily so.

Money money money

Policy-makers' concerns are always *au fond* about money. Even the (genuinely bingeing) booze-ups that are such frequent British city centre weekend attractions only really bother policy-makers because they cost so much to police and clean up – as well as driving away tourists and their wallets.* So when health authorities want politicians to listen up about the health dangers of alcohol, they often point to the cost. "Three billion pounds a year" is what booze costs Britain's NHS, are the kinds of figures regularly splashed across their morning papers.[25]

Now, like 99.9% of the population including politicians, I have no idea how that £3 billion figure was arrived at. But I'm now going to hit you with another set of figures – and 'show my working' too, as we used to have to do in Maths exams.

Most of this book has shown pretty incontrovertible evidence that, unless you go overboard on the booze, alcohol is Good News for health, preventing things like dementia, heart disease, arthritis, blahdiblah … and generally prolonging people's lives. So let's work out how much the UK NHS could *save* if everyone (including teetotallers) were to follow sensible advice about what and how much to drink, based on the medical evidence outlined in this book.

Here we go (these are all very rough and ready figures, of course):

Heart Disease
Annual Cost: £3.2 billion
Booze benefit: 25%
Saving: £0.8 billion
Diabetes

---

* On the other hand, direct and indirect alcohol costs appear to be wholly offset by the tax revenue. For example, the British government receives about £21 billion a year in alcohol-related tax income – precisely the same as alcohol is estimated to cost the nation overall (health and social costs combined).

Annual Cost: £10 billion
Booze Benefit: 20%
Saving: £2 billion

Arthritis
Annual Cost: £700 million
Booze Benefit: 85%
Saving: £0.6 billion

Dementia
Annual Cost: £20 billion
Booze Benefit: 40%
Saving: £8 billion

Total Booze Benefit: £11.6 billion

Of course, this is all very 'back of an envelope' stuff. It's shot through with problems – not least that the current NHS patient costs must already include quite a few drinkers, which logically reduces the booze savings benefit. On the other hand, the raw NHS numbers are only part of the disease costs to the wider economy in terms of disability payments, lost productivity etc. For example, heart disease is estimated to cost UK plc £29 billion, arthritis £8 billion, and diabetes £21 billion (that one rising steeply). The clinical and epidemiological evidence about alcohol has the logical but bizarre implication that, if alcohol – particularly red wine – were used as a preventive and therapeutic medicine, disease rates would fall substantially, and lives would be saved … with huge benefits to the economy.

After all, as I hinted right back in the Preface, had Big Pharma discovered red wine in their laboratories, they'd have come up with surely the most profitable – and effective – drug in history.

Overleaf: drum-roll … fanfare … for Medivin …!

This is only partly tongue-in-cheek. From any objective standpoint, the scientific evidence about alcohol in general and wine in particular overwhelmingly endorses booze's medicinal properties. Indeed, alcohol shares many of the characteristics of pharmaceutical drugs.

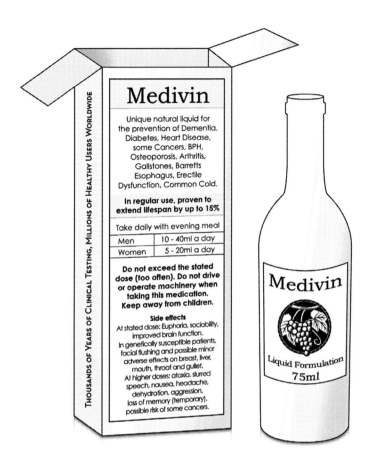

Just like a medication:

1. Alcohol has a minimum and maximum therapeutic dose. Take too little and it won't work, take too much and it may make you ill.

2. Alcohol has side-effects.* At low doses, the behavioural side-effects are (more than) benign, but they become an increasing problem at higher doses. There are also potential adverse health side-effects at high doses.

---

* Indeed, Big Pharma claims that side-effects are proof their drugs really work (but that may be nonsense).

3. Alcohol has a daily treatment regime: once a day with the evening meal. The doctor's cryptic semi-Latinate instructions to the pharmacist would say: "ON with food".*

Let's take each of those in turn.

Therapeutic Dose

The evidence is pretty clear that, in common with many medications, alcohol has different therapeutic doses depending on the condition being treated or prevented.

Heart disease seems to need at least 20 grams a day and ideally more, diabetes about 30 grams and no more, arthritis 13 grams, osteoporosis at least 28 grams, erectile dysfunction up to 40 grams, non-cancerous prostate problems over 38 grams, and dementia 20 to 30 grams.

Yes, per day.

The evidence is clear that regular alcohol consumption is indeed essential to help reduce the risk of these conditions. Studies consistently show that daily moderate drinking is the best for health.[26] This, of course, flies in the face of the medics' oft-repeated instructions to lay off the booze a few days a week. That advice does appear to be justified if you like to down skinfuls, but not if you're drinking "moderately" – a term which on the evidence of the longevity studies appears to be up to about 15 grams a day for European women and 50 grams a day for European men.[†]

Side Effects

Like all medications, alcohol does have some unhealthy side-effects, but the risks appear to be both relatively small (see Appendix One), and are far outweighed by the benefits – again like many prescription medicines.

It's the behavioural side-effects, of course, that give booze such a bad name, and of course everyone abhors alcohol-

---

* O = Omne = every; N = nocte = night (ablative case, for pedants).

† The true figures could be higher because of the under-reporting problem already discussed.

fuelled crime, road deaths, city centre mayhem, domestic violence, A&E costs etc. But I'll lay you good odds that, if it weren't for those, policy-makers wouldn't give much of a monkeys about the medical authorities' concerns over the health risks.

What's more, in less urbanised and more martial times, policy-makers would have prized those violent behavioural side-effects as sinews-stiffeners and blood-summoners in war. In fact, medieval soldiers were reputed to have been semi-ratarsed on the battlefields – and indeed booze might well have helped them survive their wounds.*

So you can't really blame alcohol for doing what it says on the tin, and the extreme end of its behavioural effects being no longer appropriate for a modern society. Alcohol is a powerful psychotropic (mood-altering) substance which in lowish doses is 'pro-social' and in higher ones anti-social.

That's the sum total of it.

The remarkable thing is that a substance which is essentially psychotropic can have such a range of health benefits – and vice versa. Quite why or how Nature, Evolution, Intelligent Design or the Lord God managed to arrange it like this is a mystery.

Daily Prevention Programme
"ON with food". Once a day with your evening meal.

Drink is best consumed on a full stomach, as food substantially slows down the absorption of alcohol. There's a valve in the stomach which regulates how quickly food nutrients (including alcohol) enter the intestine to be sucked up by the body. The fuller the stomach, the slower the nutrient release. Drinking on empty stomach means alcohol goes straight into the intestines. A Bad Idea.

Time of day. Evening is best, as we saw in Chapter 11. That's when the body's alcohol detoxifying enzymes are at peak performance, so the side-effects are bound to be

---

* A 2012 US hospital records survey counter-intuitively found that the drunker the injured patient, the better the chances of survival.

minimised and health benefits maximised. I say "bound to be" but actually I haven't a clue. I consulted Professor Alan Rosenwasser, one of the world experts on circadian rhythms and alcohol. "What's the best time of day to drink in order to maximise alcohol's health benefits and minimise its risks, Prof?" I asked. "That's a very good question" he kindly answered, "I don't know of any evidence that confining one's drinking to particular times of day influences health outcomes."

He's right; there isn't any. That's odd because there is a huge amount of research on circadian rhythms and alcohol in general; the trouble is that it's almost all focussed on alcoholism, as a 2004 survey reveals.[27] Is this a valuable use of research time (and laboratory animals), however? One wonders what purpose is served by ferreting out yet more health hazards to add to the already long litany of problems caused by alcoholism. We already know alcoholism is a no-no. End of story.

The Way Forward

It's now clear that alcohol can make a serious contribution to our health, well-being and lifespan – but like everything else in life it's also got its downsides. That's where scientific research should be concentrated: finding out how to minimise its risks and maximise its benefits. Two areas in particular are under-researched.

First, nutrition. There's quite a lot of evidence that alcohol can deplete the body of nutrients such as the B-vitamins,[28] and that boosting them may reduce some of booze's harmful effects.[29] The most important of these for drinkers appears to be folate, also known as folic acid or Vitamin B9. For example, there is good evidence that breast cancer risk is considerably reduced – and indeed can be actually reversed

– if women drinkers eat leafy vegetables or take folate supplements [30] [31]

Why haven't women been told this? Possibly because there's some evidence that Vitamin B9 can both decrease and increase cancer rates.[32] That sounds bizarre, so what's going on? Well, although folate and folic acid appear to be chemically the same substance, the former is natural and the latter synthetic, so no marks for guessing it's been discovered that the body doesn't like the synthetic type much.

That whole area needs a complete sort-out, therefore, so that women at high genetic risk of breast cancer can be advised to take the correct folate supplement if they wish to drink.

Similarly there's a compound called ubiquinone which has been found to reduce the liver damage caused by alcohol[33] – but that's hardly begun to be investigated.

There will surely be more nutrients to find; it would then simply become a matter of drinkers taking these nutrients in pill form or in their diet to get the body back to normal. At present, not a scrap of this kind of nutritional information reaches the public though.

Next genes. It's long been known that certain genetic types have a problem with alcohol, but as the science of genetics has become more sophisticated, a host of variants ("alleles") of the couple of dozen alcohol detoxifying genes have been discovered. Early indications are that some of these may have remarkably specific effects, helping to explain individual differences in people's response to booze. So it's not difficult to imagine a time when everyone who decided to drink (for fun, health or both) would first take a genetic test to discover their likely reaction to alcohol, and make the appropriate decisions.

That could be a pretty inexpensive thing to do. Already in 2013 you can get a full genetic test of your health-related genes, plus a fair sprinkling of alleles (not the alcohol ones though yet), for a mere $100.*

Genetic testing is likely to become even cheaper and more sophisticated in future. Perhaps we'll have all the genetic information about alcohol done and dusted by 2020.

But what about 2013/14? What health decisions should people make about their drinking habits on the basis of the scientific evidence currently available?

At present, national authorities' guidelines tend to be both simplistic and mildly prohibitionist, their implied message being: "we'd rather you didn't drink, but if you really must, don't drink more than x".

At the other extreme, however, some experts believe positive, evidence-based messages are more appropriate. This from alcohol researcher Professor Alfonso di Castelnuovo:

> The benefit of light to moderate drinking [is] of undoubted public health value … Heavy drinkers should be urged to cut their consumption, but people who already regularly consume low to moderate amounts of alcohol should be encouraged to continue.[34]†

The issue only comes with who should drink and who should be more circumspect, says Harvard Professor Wendy Chen, who thinks it all depends on the individual – women particularly.

> If you are someone with a family history of breast cancer but are healthy, at a good weight, exercise regularly, have a healthy diet and don't have a risk for heart disease, then you may make one decision. Another woman who has some cardiovascular risk factors and no history of breast cancer may make a different decision.[35]

But that's about as is as good as it gets at present – perhaps because, may I modestly suggest, the health evidence about alcohol as a whole has not been brought together under one roof before now. Now that's been achieved between these

---

* I had my own genes checked out by a company in California for $100 (plus far more in transatlantic postage though!)

† See reactions to this statement plus other expert opinions in Appendix Two.

covers, it might be easier for people to make up their own minds about what and how much to drink, based on their own personal health status. For example, if arthritis, heart disease or dementia run in your family, you may make one set of decisions, but if throat and breast cancer, possibly another.

All it then requires to make informed choices is to know exactly how much alcohol you're drinking. That means sensible labelling. The current 'units' and 'drinks' system is a mess – not least because very few people understand it, as a 2013 BBC straw poll demonstrated.[36]

Rather than alcohol units, what is needed is something on a par with calorie units to indicate alcohol content … we've already got it, of course: it's grams.

In fact, medical journals are now increasingly using gram measures, and shunning 'units' as being too confusing. Why not go public with the idea, and label every bottle of booze in 'grams of alcohol' content? Why should that be so difficult? Food labels are already carpeted with calorie and nutrient values, as well as impenetrable E numbers, so what's the problem with a simple number like 70 to 80 grams for a bottle of wine, 17 grams for a can of lager, 225 grams for a bottle of spirits and so on? Incidentally, as with micronutrient contents in food, wine labels could also include polyphenol content, since each wine has different concentrations of these health-promoting natural compounds.*

Talking of calories, I hear that official noises are currently being made to include calorie values on alcohol bottle labels. This is an astonishing initiative, because it is not evidence-based – or in plain language it's barking mad. As Chapter 7 amply demonstrates, the experimental and epidemiological data are clear that, for whatever reasons, alcohol 'calories' don't count.

Another barking mad initiative was floated in August 2013. Headlined by the *Daily Mail* as "Doctors call for

---

* The Pinot Noir grape, for example, has twice as many polyphenols as Cabernet or Sauvignon.

alcohol safety levels to be halved for pensioners", the story read:

> Doctors warn that heavy drinking among the elderly is a 'hidden problem'. They say that elderly drinkers' bodies are less able to cope with drinking. The Royal College of Psychiatrists wants men over 65 to be limited to 1.5 units a day and women to one unit ... Newcastle University researchers want a new recommended drinking limit for over-65s and special advice on alcohol, tailored to the needs of older people.... The researchers [said] that while the elderly may believe they have built up a tolerance to booze, alcohol can cause more damage to the ageing body.[37]

Why is this recommendation barking mad? Well, as we've already seen in Chapter 9, the evidence on alcohol and lifespan is clear that reducing alcohol intakes to those low levels would result in an increase in death rates. But more importantly it is just plain nonsense, because the science actually says that the older you get, the more you can tolerate alcohol's ill-effects and take advantage of its benefits.

That stunning fact was unequivocally established in 2002 by British scientists at the MRC Biostatistics Unit in Cambridge. They combed through the entire evidence base about alcohol and the elderly, and came to some clear 'on-balance' health recommendations:

> "Men would be advised to limit their drinking to ... 4 units a day [from] age 54 ... up to age 84, and 5 units a day over age 85. Women ... 2 units a day up to age 74, and 3 units a day over age 75."[38]

So we should increase the alcohol limits for the old, says the Medical Research Council. But do the reverse, says the University of Newcastle and the Royal College of Psychiatrists.

A mess is too polite a description for this state of affairs. It's surely absurd that expert statisticians at the British taxpayer-funded Medical Research Council can be ignored, while other less authoritative British academic bodies can blithely issue advice that is so completely contradictory to the MRC's recommendations, let alone to the broader scientific evidence.

But again, in the drive to blacken booze, anything goes.

Finally, nations should get their ducks in a row and agree on guidelines. They should take a long, cool, sober look at the evidence, stop demonising drink, and come clean about its many health benefits and very few downsides at moderate intakes.

Getting any co-ordinated international health policies in this area doesn't look too promising, however. This is how British alcohol expert, Dr Richard Harding explained to the UK Parliament in 2011 how the current mess has been created:

> World-wide recommendations on alcohol consumption show wide disparity among countries. This is in some ways surprising, given that the science is the same everywhere. But the objective of those who frame such guidance is to influence their target populations. It follows therefore that several factors then become relevant, e.g. the behaviour that is thought to be in need of change, the culture and mindset of the target population, and the kind of message that is likely to be effective. Therefore the best approach is to formulate advice firmly based on and argued from the science, but that which is also appropriate to the problems that the UK face and is likely to be effective, and not to take much notice of what other governments or health bodies recommend.

Nannystateism in a nutshell.

Ladies and gentlemen, please now raise your glasses!

The medical evidence about alcohol leads to this very clear but counter-intuitive conclusion: it is just as irresponsible to discourage people from using alcohol as it is to encourage them to drink too much.

If you don't understand that statement, you haven't understood the evidence outlined in this book, because science says that both behaviours end up with the same result: shortening your life ... whereas drinking enough to get mildly sociable but not blotto will lengthen it, by improving your overall health.

But haven't we all intuitively known that for centuries? When raising a glass, peoples everywhere, although separated in both time and space, have used exactly the same toast:

bonam sanitatem (Latin), *salud* (Spanish), *salute* (Italian), *santé* (French), *saude* (Portuguese), *Terveydeksi* (Finnish), *Gesondheid* (Afrikaans) *Sláinte* (Irish) *Nazdrowie* (Polish)... and in English:

YOUR VERY GOOD HEALTH!

Appendix One

Truths, Half-truths and Statistics

This book has thrown loads of numbers around...mainly percentage increases and decreases in the risk of getting diseases, losing weight, living longer, etc. etc.

But what do all these percentages mean in terms of our health – our ill-health in particular? After all, it's the dangers and not the benefits of booze that the medical authorities want us to be aware of.

The problem is, because we don't expire the moment a drop of alcohol passes our lips, the dangers of alcohol are always couched in terms of probabilities or possibilities of one or other health risk. This inevitably involves a bit of mathematics – or more precisely a branch of maths called statistics, and it's medical statistics that are used by the authorities as proof of alcohol's dangers.

But what do these statistics really mean in everyday health terms?

Probably because it is so emotive, the most investigated of alcohol's dangers is breast cancer. As this book went to press, there were a staggering 3,911 separate studies on the subject of women's most feared disease and their drinking habits.

Breast cancer is also a hot topic for the media medics who wish to warn everyone off drinking.

So, for lots of reasons, breast cancer is a good test case to examine the statistical science behind the claims of harm from alcohol, and a proxy for most of the other disease risks.

The Statistics of Breast Cancer

Cancer of the breast … the most scary of all cancers, as it strikes so many women – sometimes at quite a young age.

The latest UK figures show that 12,000 women a year die from it, and that a woman's chance of contracting it is roughly 1 in 8 – pretty rotten odds. After heart disease, it's the biggest cause of female premature death.

Why it's so common is a mystery. Quite a lot of it is due to a bad hand of genes, but that's by no means the whole story. So there must be some major lifestyle or environmental reasons for it being so widespread. And indeed there are, but they're almost too many to count: from being a shift worker, diabetic, overweight, sedentary, above average height or in the upper social classes, to being exposed to environmental chemicals, or consuming too few vegetables or too much booze.

The jargon term is "multifactorial", but that's by definition a very complex matter. So alcohol is an easy scapegoat – hence the medical finger being so firmly pointed at booze.

But is that really justified? Read on.

Truths

The adjective that crops up most in the medical literature to describe drinkers' risk of breast cancer is "modest". Nobody claims the risk is anything like the connection between lung cancer and smoking, for example. In fact, the figures show that drinking is roughly on a par with not taking enough exercise, [1] as both are associated with similar levels of breast cancer risk.

There's also a problem with explaining how alcohol might actually cause breast cancer. As Chapter 2 explained, the liquid itself is not cancer-causing, and neither in practice is acetaldehyde, its metabolite (except in people of Asian descent).

So quite a lot of research effort has gone into ferreting out the cause and effect connection between booze and breasts ... and after about 20 years work, medics finally think they've found it. Alcohol, they say, causes breast cancer by increasing female hormones.

How come?

Lots of distinct diseases come under the heading of breast cancer. There are two basic cancer types though, each of which hinges on whether or not the particular cancer has "receptor cells" for the two female hormones, estrogen and progesterone. Only the cancers which contain these receptor cells (so-called "hormone positive" cancers) are aggravated by female hormones; all the other breast cancers are unaffected.

Since the mid-1990s, there's been growing (albeit not wholly consistent) evidence that alcohol is associated with the hormone-positive breast cancers, but not the hormone-negative ones[2][3], implying that drinking may have a hormone-boosting effect.

So we now have a possible explanation for how alcohol might affect the breast cancer process – by increasing female hormones.

Sounds like more Bad News ... but is it? Not particularly.

For one thing, alcohol's apparent adverse effect on the hormone-positive cancers is still "modest", and for another, about 1 in 4 women now needn't worry about breast cancer and booze ever again. Really? Yes, because at least 25% of breast cancers are the hormone-negative type, and the evidence does not reveal any connection with alcohol for these cancers – however much a woman drinks. The kicker is of course that current genetic science can't say which breast cancer type any particular woman may be prone to, so at present this remains an interesting observation and no more.

On the other hand there is some Good News that can be applied today, but only if you have a strong family history of breast cancer – specifically hormone-negative breast cancer. If that's the type your mother died of, it's likely you're at risk of it too … which means that you needn't worry about booze at all, according to the evidence. That's because hormone-negative cancers don't appear to be related to alcohol, as outlined above.

However, because genetic science is still in its infancy in this area, it's simplest to give blanket information to women about the risks they run if they drink. This is what breastcancer.org tells them:

> Experts estimate that the risk of breast cancer goes up another 10% for each additional drink women regularly have each day.

Health Central says:

> For every 10g of alcohol consumed daily, breast cancer risk increases 9%

Let's examine this particular claim. 10% extra risk of breast cancer for every glass of wine or measure of spirits downed per day sounds terrifying, but is it?

Half-truths

First, let's first discover the origin of this 10% figure, and secondly do the maths to work out what it really means in practice.

Where did "10%" come from?

Partly from the chart opposite.

The chart appears in a "landmark" scientific paper called *Meta-analysis of studies of alcohol and breast cancer with consideration of the methodological issues,* written by eight high-powered academics in 2006.[4]

Each one of those dots represents one medical survey on a group of women, where the researchers connected the risk of getting a breast cancer diagnosis with the women's alcohol intake. The centre horizontal line is zero risk.

As you will see, some dots are above the centre line,

others below, meaning that in some studies drinking was found to increase the risk of a cancer diagnosis, and in others to decrease it. Examples of these 'bad news' and 'good news' breast cancer studies were given in Chapters 2 and 12.

Two things are immediately striking about this chart: how close to zero many of these dots are, and how scattered they are (in fact, it's called a "scatter plot"). Indeed, they would appear to be almost random. However, computers are damn clever, as we all know, so it probably takes just a few key presses to see if there's any sense to be made out of this apparent randomness.

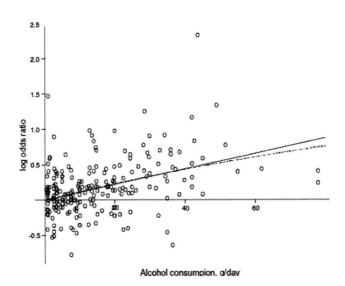

Scatter plot of the log odds ratios of the risk of breast cancer associated with alcoholic consumption. Reproduced by permission from Key J et al. *Cancer Causes & Control* (2006) 17: 759–70.

That's almost certainly how that gently rising straight line across the page was produced. It's this kind of computer-generated analysis that is used to support the "one drink a day raises your risk of breast cancer by 10%" statement.

Now of course, what's computer determined isn't necessarily biologically determined. If there are consistently "heterogeneous" (i.e inconsistent) findings, as the breast cancer/alcohol data demonstrate, biological logic rather than computer logic suggests that the connection between the two might be somewhat tenuous.

Statistics

But what's the extra breast cancer risk from alcohol anyway?

In statistics, there are two types of risk: Relative and Absolute. What's the difference, and why is that important?

Here's an everyday example: the UK National Lottery. As everyone knows, there is a very remote chance of winning it – 1 in 14 million.

That's if you buy 1 ticket. However, if you buy 2 tickets, your odds reduce to 1 in 7 million, and if you buy 3 tickets to 4.6 million. Your Absolute Odds or Risk of winning still remain millions to one therefore, but your Relative Odds or Risk of winning has zoomed up. Here's a chart of what these different chances of winning the Lottery look like.

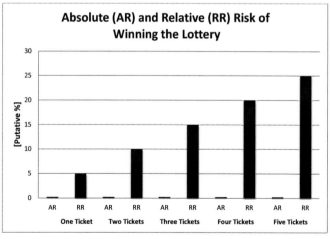

Absolute and Relative Risk of Winning the Lottery by ticket purchases

For each lottery ticket you buy, your Relative Risk of winning climbs steeply, but your Absolute Risk remains essentially the same – almost zero.

The same basic principle applies to health statistics such as alcohol and breast cancer. When medical studies – or the medical authorities - report their findings on alcohol, they invariably express them in terms of Relative Risk. So, when they say women have a 10% extra risk of breast cancer every time they take a drink, it's a Relative not an Absolute Risk.

Sadly, women already have quite a high Absolute Risk of getting breast cancer – simply by virtue of being alive and female. So, what does having a drink mean to their Absolute Risk in Lottery-type terms?

Let's take an everyday example of a woman who drinks half a bottle of wine (40 grams of alcohol) a day. According to the authorities, she will raise her risk of breast cancer by 4 times 10% = 40%. That's a Relative Risk, of course, not an Absolute Risk.

Here's a graph of what the two risks look like:

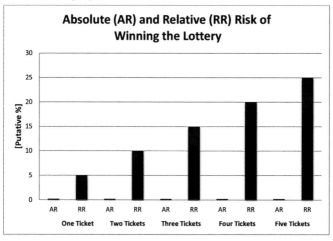

Absolute and Relative Risk of getting breast cancer

Assuming drinking 40 grams of alcohol a day raises the

Relative Risk of getting breast cancer by 40%,* the increase in Absolute Risk is about a tenth of that. By the same token, drinking 10 grams a day results in an extra risk not of 10% but of 1.2%

This is how the sums are done.

> 1. We know – courtesy of Cancer Research UK – that women have an overall lifetime risk of 1 in 8 of getting breast cancer.
>
> 2. We also know that about 50% of UK women are regular drinkers.†
>
> 3. Therefore, of the 1 in 8 women who get breast cancer, some will be drinkers, some not. That subtly shifts the overall statistics.
>
> 4. 1 in 8 women getting breast cancer means that every woman has a baseline 12.5 % Absolute Risk of the disease. Assuming 50% of the women who get the cancer are drinkers and the rest are teetotal, that 12.5% translates into a risk for non-drinkers of 10.4%, and a risk for drinkers of 14.6% – i.e. an extra 4.2% risk compared to teetotallers, but only an extra 2.1% risk over the baseline 12.5%.

The breast cancer statistics get even more complicated (but relevant for lifestyle choices) if a woman's age is taken into account.[5] Before age 50, her breast cancer risk is pretty low – roughly 2%. Assuming a 40% extra relative risk if she drinks 40 grams a day, her Absolute Risk rises to 2.3% – i.e. by just 0.3%.

After age 50, breast cancer Absolute Risk climbs sharply - to roughly 6%. Again, assuming a 40% relative risk, the Absolute Risk now rises to 7%. However, by that time of her life, a woman starts to be at risk of diseases other than breast

---

*   Incidentally, 40% is somewhat higher than the average risk figure in breast cancer studies.

†   The precise percentage makes little difference to the calculations

cancer – diabetes, stroke, dementia and particularly heart disease … and that substantially alters the risk equation, because at that age:

> Heart disease deaths are nine times more frequent than breast cancer deaths, and stroke is three or four times more common. Hence, even for a slight increase in the risk of breast cancer for alcohol intake, on average a post-menopausal woman who stops any alcohol intake in order to lower her risk of breast cancer may be increasing her risk of other diseases, and the net effect may be a shorter lifespan.[6]

Appendix Two

What should Joe Public be told?

1. Professional responses* to the proposal that:

"Heavy drinkers should be urged to cut their consumption, but people who already regularly consume low to moderate amounts of alcohol should be encouraged to continue."

Professor Maurizio Ponz de Leon, University of Modena, Italy:

I do not want to dispute the scientific background of this contention, which could be well-grounded, but I remain unconvinced of the evidence. The message seems to me hazardous and extremely dangerous to promote to the general population, for the following reasons at least:

1. People may be unable to distinguish between low-to-moderate and high consumption of wine, beer or spirits. Moreover, alcohol metabolism may differ remarkably from one person to another. In current clinical practice, we observe severe liver or gastric damage associated with relatively low volumes of alcohol (especially in women), whereas other patients may tolerate without any apparent explanation large amounts of alcohol.

2. It offers a "moral" justification for drinking, even if in low-to- moderate amounts.

3. If "people who are already regular light-to-moderate alcohol consumers should be encouraged to continue", by the same token, we should encourage the abstemious to drink low-to-moderate amounts of alcohol, in order to lower

---

* These have been edited for clarity and brevity.

HDL, to inhibit platelet aggregation and so on. Are we truly at the point of prescribing alcohol consumption in order to reduce the risk of stroke and coronary damage?

More studies are needed before we can give sensible recommendations on alcohol consumption to the general population. Even when further evidence of a beneficial effort may be obtained, I would suggest that we use prudence in dispensing indications for common drinks such as wine, beer or spirits; these are part of our culture and usually make for some joy in our lives, but can also contribute to causing much disease and suffering.[1]

Dr Alfonso Di Castelnuovo, University of Campobasso, Italy:

What should we advise an adult who regularly drinks a glass of wine during meals: to stop drinking? Why? What is the scientific evidence to support such negative advice? We are not convinced that many people might be unable to distinguish between low-to-moderate and high doses of wine beer or spirits; we refute such a 'paternalistic' attitude, and cannot believe that this is a sufficient argument to disregard scientific evidence. Besides alcohol, there are plenty of situations in which moderation is better than excess or abstention (e.g., the protective effect of low-dose aspirin in secondary cardiovascular risk prevention). The positive effect of sleeping pills cannot be obscured by the fact that some use an excess of these pills and harm themselves. We agree that great caution has to be taken when speaking about alcohol and health, but strongly believe that a scientific approach should always prevail over ideological prejudice.[2]

Professor Ramon Estruch, University of Barcelona, Spain:

High alcohol intake may be a cause of several chronic diseases, as well as social and labour problems. Thus, we must be cautious when recommending low-to-moderate alcohol consumption to the overall population. However, we cannot forget the scientific evidence supporting the beneficial effects of moderate alcohol/wine intake on cardiovascular disease, some types of cancer and other degenerative diseases. Cardiovascular disease continues to be the main cause of death in developed and developing countries, and we have to fight against it with all the weapons available. There is increasing evidence for a beneficial effect of the Mediterranean diet on the prevention of cardiovascular disease, and wine is one of the traditional components of this food pattern. In our experience, most people are able to distinguish between low-to-moderate wine consumption and a high amount of alcohol intake. Up to now, no randomised controlled trial has ever been conducted to assess to what extent moderate alcohol consumption offers greater benefits than complete alcohol abstinence, so we are not allowed to recommend moderate alcohol consumption to 'teetotallers', and we have to be very cautious with our recommendations to the overall population.[3]

Professor R. Curtis Ellison, Boston University School of Medicine, USA:

Abraham Lincoln said: 'The problems with alcohol in this country relate not to the use of a bad thing, but to the abuse of a good thing.' The finest moral rationale for prevention-oriented public health activity should be informing people, and it should not be based on 'paternalism' ("we know what is best for you"). We have already seen examples of sound scientific information about alcohol being sacrificed in order to be "politically correct."* There are certain people

---

* This refers to a report from the celebrated Framingham Heart Study, which found after 24 years research that teetotallers had more coronary heart disease than drinkers. However, the study had been funded by the National Institute of Health which ordered the researchers to "remove all references to alcohol" from their report, because "an article which openly invites the encouragement of undertaking drinking with the implication of preventing CHD would be scientifically misleading and socially

who should not drink at all (including former abusers of drugs or alcohol, people with certain medical conditions, or children and adolescents), so there can never be a general recommendation for everybody to consume alcohol. On the other hand, we should not withhold from our patients and the public scientifically sound and balanced data on alcohol and health.[4]

Professor Harvey Finkel, Boston University Medical Center, USA:

Physicians must communicate fully with their patients. Alcohol (chiefly wine) should be used to enrich life, not necessarily to medicate it.[5]

Professor Erik Skovenborg, Scandinavian Medical Alcohol Board, Denmark:

Problems can arise when an 'expert' states that he is unconvinced by the evidence when he is not a real expert in the field of alcohol and health. Professor de Leon and others insist that randomised, prospective clinical studies are needed before sensible recommendations about alcohol consumptions can be made. However, such investigations have never been done regarding exercise, diet, weight reduction, smoking, etc., because such studies would either be unethical, extremely costly, or extremely difficult to perform."[6]

Drs Maritha J. Kotze & David Van Velden, University of Stellenbosch, South Africa:

The debate on the health benefits of low to moderate alcohol consumption must take into consideration genetic predisposition for certain diseases. Molecular biology has

undesirable in view of the major health problem of alcoholism that already exists in the country. If you must say something about alcohol, say it has no effect." Rather than lie, the researchers decided not to publish the data. [Reported in Seltzer CC (1997). "Conflicts of interest" and "political science." *J Clin Epidemiol* 50:627–9]

made it possible for us to identify certain individuals who may not benefit from alcohol consumption. It is not possible to formulate general guidelines without recognising the fact that people react differently to drugs. Some medications meant to treat disease are also toxic to people if their bodies cannot metabolise the drug, and alcohol is no different. [7]

Professor Ulrich Keil, University of Münster, Germany:

When I submitted the first paper with German data on alcohol consumption and its relation to CHD and total mortality in a beer drinking population of southern Germany, I was afraid that it would not be accepted because I argued in this paper that the protective effect of alcohol on CHD was almost as strong as the negative effect of smoking on CHD.

In the same year another paper based on 490,000 men and women clearly showed that those smoked but didn't drink had the highest all-cause mortality, while non-smoking drinkers had the lowest; the other groupings were in between.

These studies appeared more than a decade ago, but the old arguments of 'I do not believe' are repeated again and again by certain groups or individuals – some because of conflicts of interest, political science, or paternalism, others by colleagues who are afraid of the 'devil alcohol.'[8]

Dr Tedd Goldfinger, University of Arizona, USA:

I reject the notion Dr de Leon projects that we consider, or not consider, alcohol as a medication. As clinicians, we not only prescribe medications, but also discuss healthy lifestyle choices with our patients so as to promote better health and longevity. Would he consider as "medications" fresh fish, green vegetables, and fruit and nuts, all of which contribute to a healthy and longer life?[9]

Dr Dee Blackhurst, University of Cape Town Health, South Africa:

In my experience, social pressures for excessive

consumption of alcohol to which adolescents and young adults are subjected are far greater than any pressure that could be exerted by a paper in a medical journal, even if the findings were reported in the mass media. However, older people who might be concerned about health issues and who have survived the earlier social pressures without indulging in alcohol abuse are very likely to be sensible enough to understand the meaning of moderate consumption of alcohol. Therefore it seems to me that the comments by Dr de Leon do not have much practical relevance.[10]

Professor Arthur Klatsky, Kaiser Permanente Division of Research, USA:

Most people know very well what the difference is between light to moderate drinking and binge or excessive drinking. While some patients may rationalise their heavy drinking because of its purported health effects, I have yet to find someone who had developed alcohol abuse because of messages about the health effects of moderate drinking. Doctors have a solemn duty to tell the truth about alcohol consumption, as they understand it, to all of their patients.[11]

2. Extracts from evidence to UK Parliament[12]

HOUSE OF COMMONS
Oral evidence taken before the
Health and Science & Technology Committees
October 2011 and April 2012

Sir Ian Gilmore, Alcohol Health Alliance, UK:

There has been a lot of work looking at the supposed beneficial effects or less detrimental effects of different beverages – the health benefits of red wine as opposed to other colours of wine, and so on. You can find some research to suit whatever case you want to put on the day. The reason is that there is probably virtually no difference. What really matters to your body is the amount of alcohol you take in. We know that there are incredible innate differences between individuals in the way their bodies handle alcohol and there may well be individual differences in the way we handle different sorts of alcohol, but the bottom line, so far as your body is concerned, is how much alcohol you have taken in, both acutely in order to get drunk and chronically to sustain permanent damage.

Dr Richard Harding, Member of the '1995 Interdepartmental Working Group on Sensible Drinking':

Looking at what I regard as the beneficial effects of moderate consumption on coronary heart disease, through to dementia and osteoporosis and so on, which are the diseases of ageing, it seems that there are considerable public health benefits to be gained in that age group by sensible consumption.

Gilmore: Some of us are less taken with that link, with the protection from cardio-vascular disease given by alcohol. There probably is an effect, but it does not affect the main age group that is damaged by alcohol. The peak deaths from alcohol are among 45 to 65-year-olds, who are in the most productive phase of their lives. There are serious scientists who still believe that the apparent cardio-vascular benefits are spurious. I am not going down that line, but I believe it is overplayed as a benefit.

Professor Nick Heather, Alcohol Research UK:

The main difficulty is what are known technically as confounds, i.e. unknown factors that might influence the relationship between drinking and morality, heart disease and so on. It is known as the "sick quitter" hypothesis; in other words, the objection is that people saying that they are abstainers may be abstaining because they have an alcohol problem or are unwell. The other kind of possible confound, which is now quite easy to understand, is that the moderate drinkers at the bottom of the J-shaped curve are in fact healthy, well-living people, and that low alcohol consumption is not so much a cause of longevity as a marker of a health lifestyle.

Harding: I would not agree with that. It seems to me that the evidence has got stronger over the years. The "sick quitter" hypothesis is that the abstainers are unwell and therefore have a higher rate of disease. However, some studies have been large enough to take them out, yet when you omit the sick quitters and lifetime abstainers you still see the effect. In many studies, the confounding factor has been taken care of.

Dr Marsha Morgan, Institute of Alcohol Studies

The biggest body of evidence that we have relates to the cardio-protective effect. I emphasise that, if there were to be a cardio-protective effect, it would selectively be found in middle-aged men and post-menopausal women, and you do not gain that protective effect by drinking done before then; it is an effect at the time. You cannot justify someone in that age group who does not drink starting to drink for the cardio-protective effect. After all, it is still within guidelines at between one and two units.

The two other areas where there have been alleged protective effects from the recent Million Women Study are in the development of diabetes and possibly cancers. However, there is not as strong an evidence base as that for the cardio-protective effect. Much more important, since the guidelines were last considered in 1995, is the detrimental effect of alcohol and the cancer risk, particularly for breast cancer in women, a quite significant risk of cancer of the oropharynx, larynx and oesophagus, cancers among people who already have liver damage, and to a degree some early evidence on bowel cancer. As far as I am concerned, those detrimental effects overwhelm any potential benefit that there might be on diabetes.

Harding: These are the categories of evidence that have emerged since 1995.

The first was the finding that frequency of drinking is as important as the amount consumed, within the moderate consumption band. It is clear that drinkers get more benefit from not bingeing in any way, and from keeping consumption small and moderate. A nice study came out a couple of years ago comparing drinking levels in Northern Ireland and France. I believe that in France it was an average of 30 grams a day, and in Belfast it was 20 grams a day. However, because the pattern of drinking was less frequent in Belfast, the overall health outcome was worse there than it was in France, where they had a healthier pattern of drinking. The second was the evidence of the cardio-protective effect, which has already been mentioned. The evidence *[of benefit]* for Type 2 diabetes was pretty clear in 1995, but it has been reinforced by further studies. There seems to be less osteoporosis in older people for moderate drinkers compared to abstainers, leading to an increase in bone mineral density and fewer fractures – an improvement of about 20%. Among older consumers there seems to be a reduced risk of dementia. A lot of work has been done on the effect of alcohol on cognitive function; again, there is about a 20% reduction for moderate drinkers over abstainers.

My colleague is correct that quite a lot of work has been done on cancer. The Million Women Study referred to showed an increased risk of breast cancer, and cancers of the oral cavity, the oesophagus and the larynx, which was expected, but a decreased risk of non-Hodgkin's lymphoma, thyroid and renal carcinoma. The overall risk of cancer to women in that group was lower in moderate consumers than in abstainers. When it got to between 7 and 14 drinks a week, however, it was about the same.

I urge the Committee to keep a sense of perspective. With breast cancer there seems to be an increasing risk of about 5% to 10% per drink per day. If a woman aged 20 has a lifetime risk, let us say, of 20% of getting breast cancer before the age of 75, a drink per day would increase that risk to 21% or 22%. Up to the menopause, the risk is much lower – say 5% or 10%. If it was 5%, the increased risk would be 5.5%. If it was 10%, the increased risk would be 11%. After the menopause, women are exposed to the risk of cardio-vascular diseases; before that they are protected by their hormones. The benefit that they gain from moderate consumption after the menopause would outweigh any increased risk of cancer. There is a risk, but on balance the data show that if they wish to consume alcohol for health reasons the net effect is beneficial.

Heather: My advice is that under no circumstances should the Committee recommend that the guidelines are increased. That would be inimical to the health of the nation and wrong on the best scientific evidence. There is no case for increasing them.

Gilmore: I would go with Professor Heather. As someone who looks after patients with liver disease who sees hospital admissions rising year on year and now topping one million, a recommendation to increase the limits would be swimming against the tide of harm that we see in our hospitals every day. The most important thing is that we should have a single, consistent message not only for the general public but for the health professionals, so that they know what message they should be conveying when they see their patients.

3. Extracts from *Think About Drink; there's more to a drink than you think*.[13]

A 16 page, 5 colour, 21x15 cms pamphlet on 120 g coated paper, published by Britain's Health Education Authority in 1996.

"Alcohol is a positive part of life for most people.

Alcohol is something to be enjoyed and most of the time, drinking alcohol doesn't cause any problems.

For men over 40, there can be positive health benefits from drinking moderate amounts of alcohol.

For women who have been through the menopause, there can be positive health benefits from drinking moderate amounts of alcohol.

The Health Benefits

Studies have shown that people who regularly drink small amounts of alcohol tend to live longer than people who don't drink at all. The main reason is that alcohol gives protection against the development of coronary heart disease. Alcohol influences the amount of cholesterol carried in the bloodstream and also makes it less likely that clots will form.

It seems that you can't build up protection from coronary heart disease in earlier years. The protective effect is only significant when people reach a stage in life when they are at risk of coronary heart disease. For men, this means once you're over the age of 40. For women, it's after the menopause.

The major part of the health benefit can be obtained at levels as low a 1 unit a day, with the maximum health advantage lying between 1 and 2 units a day. No additional overall benefit comes from drinking more than 2 units a day.

The benefits come from drinking small amounts of alcohol fairly regularly, so drinking large amounts intermittently (eg. only at weekends) doesn't have as much benefit as drinking 1 unit a day.

There is no clear evidence that any one type of drink (eg. red wine) gives any more protection than any other type of drink.* So if you prefer beer or spirits, you can still get the benefits.

There are many reasons why people choose not to drink alcohol. If you don't wish to drink alcohol, no-one is going to suggest that you have to start now. There are other things you can do to reduce your risk of coronary heart disease

Children are aware of alcohol at an early age. Between the age of 10 and 13, most children have had their first alcohol drink. This introduction to alcohol usually takes place at home with parents letting children have an odd sip or a small glass on a special occasion.

Alcohol can be a source of pleasure and enjoyment. By following the guidelines in this leaflet you can make sure that you can drink alcohol without putting yourself or others at risk."

This glossily produced pamphlet was the world's first (and to date only) official public health document to reveal the health benefits of alcohol. However, it appears never to have been distributed. Apart from the one copy retained in the British Library, the entire print run seems to have vanished into thin air.

---

* As this book shows, subsequent scientific research has added many more diseases that alcohol protects against, and revealed the particular benefits of wine.

References

Chapter 1

1   Royal College of Physicians (1987) Report: Alcohol — a great and growing evil: the medical consequences of alcohol abuse. Royal College of Physicians, London.

2   Royal College of Physicians and British Paediatric Association (1995) Report of a Joint Working Party: Alcohol and the young. Royal College of Physicians, London.

3   Royal College of Psychiatrists and Royal College of General Practitioners (1995) Report of a Joint Working Party: Alcohol and the heart in perspective: sensible drinking reaffirmed. Royal College of Physicians, London.

4   Royal College of Physicians (2001) Report of a Working Party: Alcohol — can the NHS afford it? Recommendations for a coherent alcohol strategy for hospitals. Royal College of Physicians, London.

5   Alcohol-use disorders – preventing the development of hazardous and harmful drinking. NICE Public health guidance, PH24. June 2010.

6   Richard Smith. "Battling over safe alcohol limits" *BMJ blogs* 14 Nov, 2011.

7   *The Times*, 20 Oct, 2007.

8   ICAP Reports No.14, December 2003.

9   ICAP Reports No.5, September 1998.

Chapter 2

1   Alcohol Concern Press Release, 12 October 2012.

2   "NHS Choices. Your health, your choices" webpage.

3   WCRF/AICR Food, Nutrition, Physical Activity, and the Prevention of Cancer: a Global Perspective. AICR: Washington, DC; 2007

4   Park JY et al. (2010). Alcohol intake and risk of colorectal cancer: Results from the UK Dietary Cohort Consortium *Br J Cancer.* 2010 August 24; 103 (5): 747–756.

5   Ferrari, P et al. (2007). Lifetime and baseline alcohol intake and risk of colon and rectal cancers in the European prospective investigation into cancer and nutrition (EPIC). *International Journal of Cancer,* 121(9), 2065–2072.

6   Hjartåker A et al. (2013) Subsite-Specific Dietary Risk Factors for

Colorectal Cancer: A Review of Cohort Studies *J Oncol.* 2013; 2013: 703854. Published online 2013 March 12. doi: 10.1155/2013/703854

7   Cho E et al. (2004) Alcohol intake and colorectal cancer: a pooled analysis of 8 cohort studies. *Ann Intern Med.* Apr 20; 140 (8): 603–13.

8   Park, JY et al. (2009). Baseline alcohol consumption, type of alcoholic beverage and risk of colorectal cancer in the European Prospective Investigation into Cancer and Nutrition-Norfolk study. *Cancer Epidemiology,* 33(5), 347–54.

9   Crockett, SD et al. (2011). Inverse relationship between moderate alcohol intake and rectal cancer: analysis of the North Carolina Colon Cancer Study. *Diseases of the colon and rectum,* 54(7), 887.

10   Gapstur SM et al. (1994).Alcohol consumption and colon and rectal cancer in postmenopausal women. *Int J Epidemiol.* Feb; 23 (1): 50–7.

11   Ajmo JL at al. (2008) Resveratrol alleviates alcoholic fatty liver in mice *Am J Physiol Gastrointest Liver Physiol* 295: G833–G842 .

12   Bishayee A et al. 2010 Resveratrol in the chemoprevention and treatment of hepatocellular carcinoma. *Cancer Treat Rev* 36 (1): 43–53.

13   Seitz HK, Pöschl, G and Simanowski, UA. (1998). Alcohol and Cancer. In Recent Developments in Alcoholism: *The Consequences of Alcoholism,* Galanter, M., ed., pp. 67–96. Plenum Press, New York, London.

14   BBC *Panorama,* 20 Feb 2012.

15   Becker U et al. (1996) Prediction of risk of liver disease by alcohol intake, sex and age: a prospective population study. *Hepatology* 23: 1025–29.

16   Sørensen TI et al. (1984) Prospective evaluation of alcohol abuse and alcoholic liver injury in men as predictors of development of cirrhosis *Lancet* 4; 2 (8397): 241–4.

17   Bellentani S (1997) Drinking habits as cofactors of risk for alcohol induced liver damage *Gut*; 41: 845–50.

18   Stokkeland K et al. (2008) Different drinking patterns for women and men with alcohol dependence with and without alcoholic cirrhosis *Alcohol;* 43: 39–45.

19   Monzoni A et al. (2001) Genetic determinants of ethanol-induced liver damage *Mol Med*; 7 (4): 255–62.

20   Järveläinen HA et al. (2001).Promoter polymorphism of the CD14 endotoxin receptor gene as a risk factor for alcoholic liver disease. *Hepatology*; 33 (5): 1148–53.

21   Stroffolini T et al. (2010) Interaction of alcohol intake and cofactors on the risk of cirrhosis. *Liver Int.* 30 (6): 867–70.

22   Lieber CS (2003) Relationships between nutrition, alcohol use, and liver disease. *Alcohol Res Health.* 2003; 27 (3): 220–31.

23   Dunn W et al. (2012) Modest alcohol consumption is associated with decreased prevalence of steatohepatitis in patients with non-alcoholic fatty liver disease (NAFLD).*J Hepatol.*; 57 (2): 384–91.

24   Mueller S et al. (2009) Alcoholic liver disease and hepatitis C: a frequently underestimated combination. *World J Gastroenterol.* 28; 15 (28): 3462–71.

25   La Vecchia C, Zhang ZF, Altieri A (2008) Alcohol and laryngeal cancer: an update *Eur J Cancer Prev.* 17 (2): 116–24.

26   Kobo A et al. (2009). Alcohol types and sociodemographic characteristics as risk factors for Barrett's esophagus *Gastroenterology.* 136 (3): 806–15.

27   Thrift AP et al. (2011). Lifetime alcohol consumption and risk of Barrett's esophagus. *American Journal of Gastroenterology,* 106 (7), 1220–1230.

28   Islami F et al (2011) Alcohol drinking and esophageal squamous cell carcinoma with focus on light-drinkers and never-smokers: a systematic review and meta-analysis. *Int J Cancer.* 2011 Nov 15; 129 (10): 2473–84.

29   Blot WJ, McLaughlin JK (1999) The changing epidemiology of esophageal cancer. *Semin Oncol* 26 (5 Suppl 15): 2–8.

30   *NIAAA* No. 21 PH 345 July 1993.

31   Scientists rethink alcohol/breast cancer relationship *NIAAA* 16 Oct 2012.

32   Chen WY et al. (2011) Moderate alcohol consumption during adult life, drinking patterns, and breast cancer risk. *JAMA*; 306: 1884–1890.

33   Terry MB et al. (2006) Lifetime alcohol intake and breast cancer risk. *Ann Epidemiol.* Mar; 16 (3): 230–40.

34   Mørch LS et al. (2007). Alcohol drinking, consumption patterns and breast cancer among Danish nurses: a cohort study. *European Journal of Public Health,* 17 (6), 624–9.

35   Smith-Warner SA et al. (1998). Alcohol and breast cancer in women. A pooled analysis of cohort studies. *JAMA*; 279: 535–40.

36   Longnecker MP et al.(1995) Risk of breast cancer in relation to lifetime alcohol consumption. *J Natl Cancer Inst*; 87: 923–9.

37   Tonnesen H et al. (1994) Cancer morbidity in alcohol abusers. *Br J Cancer*; 69 (2): 327–32.

38   Kuper H et al. (2000) Alcohol and Breast Cancer risk: the alcoholism paradox *British Journal of Cancer*; 83 (7): 949–51.

39   Barnett GC et al. (2008). Risk factors for the incidence of breast cancer: do they affect survival from the disease? *J Clin Oncol.* 2008 Jul 10; 26 (20): 3310–6.

40   Bessaoud F, Daurès JP (2008) Patterns of alcohol (especially wine) consumption and breast cancer risk: a case-control study among a

population in Southern France. *Ann Epidemiol.*; Jun 18 (6) :467–75.

41   Schütze M et al. (2011). Alcohol attributable burden of incidence of cancer in eight European countries based on results from prospective cohort study. *British Medical Journal*, 342. d1584.

42   Hackney JF, Engelman RW, Good RA (1992) Ethanol calories do not enhance breast cancer in isocalorically fed C3H/Ou mice. *Nutr Cancer.* 1992; 18 (3): 245–53.

43   Watabiki T et al. (2000) Long-term ethanol consumption in ICR mice causes mammary tumor in females and liver fibrosis in males. *Alcohol Clin Exp Res* 24: 117S–122S.

44   Brooks PJ, Zakhari S (2013) Moderate Alcohol Consumption and Breast Cancer in Women: From Epidemiology to Mechanisms and Interventions, *Alcohol Clin Exp Res,* Vol 37, No 1: pp 23–30.

45   Seitz HK et al. (2012) Epidemiology and Pathophysiology of Alcohol and Breast Cancer: Update 2012 *Alcohol and Alcoholism* Vol. 47, No. 3: 204–12.

46   Hong J et al. (2010) Alcohol consumption promotes mammary tumor growth and insulin sensitivity. *Cancer Lett.* August 28; 294 (2): 229–35.

47   *Boston University Critique* 089: Combination of hormone treatments and alcohol consumption influences the risk of breast cancer in women. 29 August 2012.

48   Smith-Warner SA et al. (1998) Alcohol and breast cancer in women: a pooled analysis of cohort studies. *JAMA.* 18; 279 (7): 535–40 49 Hunter DJ, Willett WC (1996) Nutrition and breast cancer. *Cancer Causes Control.* 1996 Jan; 7 (1): 56–68.

50   Chen WY et al. (2011) Moderate alcohol consumption during adult life, drinking patterns, and breast cancer risk. *JAMA.* November 2; 306 (17): 1884–90.

51   Lee JE et al. (2007) Alcohol intake and renal cell cancer in a pooled analysis of 12 prospective studies *J Natl Cancer Inst.* 16; 99 (10): 801–10.

52   Pelucchi C, et al. (2008) Alcohol consumption and renal cell cancer risk in two Italian case-control studies *Ann Oncol.* 19 (5): 1003–8.

53   Tramacere I et al. (2012) A meta-analysis on alcohol drinking and gastric cancer risk *Ann Oncol.* 23 (1): 28–36.]

54   Barstad B et al. (2005) Intake of wine, beer and spirits and risk of gastric cancer *Eur J Cancer Prev.*14 (3): 239–43.

55   Duell EJ et al. (2011).Alcohol consumption and gastric cancer risk in the European Prospective Investigation into Cancer and Nutrition (EPIC) cohort *Am J Clin Nutr* 2011; 94: 1266–75.

56   Meinhold CL (2009) Alcohol intake and risk of thyroid cancer in the NIH-AARP Diet and Health Study *Br J Cancer.* 3; 101 (9): 1630–4.

57   Arranz S et al. (2012). Wine, beer, alcohol and polyphenols on cardiovascular disease and cancer. *Nutrients*, 4 (7), 759–81.

58   US Food and Drug Administration, Code of Federal Regulations, Title 21, Volume 3, April 1, 2006.

59   Acetaldehyde (CAS NO. 75–07–0) U.S. Environmental Protection Agency August 1994.

60   *Ibid.*

61   Soffritti M et al. (2002). Results of Long⊠Term Experimental Studies on the Carcinogenicity of Formaldehyde and Acetaldehyde in Rats. *Annals of the New York Academy of Sciences,* 982 (1), 87–105.

62   Balbo S et al. (2012). Kinetics of DNA adduct formation in the oral cavity after drinking alcohol. *Cancer Epidemiol Biomarkers Prev.*; 1(4): 601–8.

63   *Daily Mail* 23 August 2012.

64   Garaycoechea JI et al (2012) Genotoxic consequences of endogenous aldehydes on mouse haematopoietic stem cell function. *Nature.* 27; 489 (7417): 571–5.

65   *Nature* podcast 7 July 2011.

66   Patra J et al. (2010) Alcohol consumption and the risk of morbidity and mortality for different stroke types – a systematic review and meta-analysis *BMC Public Health* 10: 258.

67   Klatsky AL et al. (1977). Alcohol consumption and blood pressure: Kaiser-Permanente multiphasic health examination data. *New England Journal of Medicine,* 296 (21), 1194–1200.

68   Klatsky AL (2004) Alcohol-associated hypertension. *Hypertension* 44: 805–06.

69   Irving HM, Samokhvalov AV, Rehm J. (2009). Alcohol as a risk factor for pancreatitis. A systematic review and meta-analysis. *Jop,* 10 (4), 387.

70   Henderson J, Kesmodel U, Gray R (2007) Systematic review of the fetal effects of prenatal binge-drinking *J Epidemiol Community Health* 61: 1069–73.

71   Thomas JD, Warren KR Hewitt BG (undated) Fetal Alcohol Spectrum Disorders: From Research to Policy, *NIAAA.*

72   *Ibid.*

73   Bakker R et al. (2010). Associations of light and moderate maternal alcohol consumption with fetal growth characteristics in different periods of pregnancy: The Generation R Study. *International Journal of Epidemiology,* 39 (3), 777–89.

Chapter 3

1   Mukamal KJ, Rimm EB (2001) Alcohol's Effects on the Risk for

Coronary Heart Disease. *Alcohol Research and Health*, *25*(4), 255–62

2   Joline WJ et al. (2007) Alcohol Consumption and Risk for Coronary Heart Disease among Men with Hypertension. *Annals of Internal Medicine.* Jan;146(1): 10–19.

3   Doll R et al. (1994). Mortality in relation to consumption of alcohol: 13 years' observations on male British doctors. *British Medical Journal*, *309*(6959), 911.

4   Rimm EB et al. (1999) Moderate alcohol intake and lower risk of coronary heart disease: meta-analysis of effects on lipids and haemostatic factors. *British Medical Journal* 319.7224 (1999): 1523.

5   Pearson TA (1996). Alcohol and heart disease. *Circulation*, *94*(11), 3023–25.

6   Iestra JA et al. (2005). Effect Size Estimates of Lifestyle and Dietary Changes on All-Cause Mortality in Coronary Artery Disease Patients A Systematic Review. *Circulation*, *112*(6), 924–34.

7   Thun M J et al. (1997). Alcohol consumption and mortality among middle-aged and elderly US adults. *New England Journal of Medicine*, *337*(24), 1705–14.

8   Brien SE et al. (2011). Effect of alcohol consumption on biological markers associated with risk of coronary heart disease: systematic review and meta-analysis of interventional studies. *BMJ*; 342: d636

9   Stampfer MJ et al. (1991). A prospective study of cholesterol, apolipoproteins, and the risk of myocardial infarction. *New England Journal of Medicine*, 325(6), 373–81.

10   Brien SE, op.cit.

11   Mukamal KJ et al. (2004). Alcohol consumption and inflammatory markers in older adults: the Cardiovascular Health Study. *Atherosclerosis*, *173*(1), 79–87

12   Rimm EB, Klatsky A, Grobbee D, Stampfer MJ (1996). Review of moderate alcohol consumption and reduced risk of coronary heart disease: is the effect due to beer, wine, or spirits?. *BMJ*, *312*(7033), 731–36.

13   Rimm EB, Williams P, Fosher K, Criqui M, Stampfer MJ (1999). Moderate alcohol intake and lower risk of coronary heart disease: meta-analysis of effects on lipids and haemostatic factors. *BMJ,* 319 (7224), 1523; and Ellison RC. (2005) Importance of pattern of alcohol consumption. *Circulation.* Dec 20; 112 (25): 3818–9.

14   Wouters S, Marshall R, Yee RL, Jackson R. (2000). Is the apparent cardioprotective effect of recent alcohol consumption due to confounding by prodromal symptoms? *American Journal of Epidemiology*, 151 (12), 1189–93.

15   An Update on Alcohol and Health, Dr R. Curtis Ellison, *AIM Digest*, April 2008

16   Mukamal KJ et al. (2005). Alcohol consumption and platelet activation and aggregation among women and men: the Framingham Offspring Study. *Alcoholism: Clinical and Experimental Research,* 29 (10), 1906–12.

17   Corrao G et al. (2000) Alcohol and coronary heart disease: a meta-analysis *Addiction* Oct; 95 (10): 1505–23.

18   Le Strat Y, Gorwood P (2011) Hazardous drinking is associated with a lower risk of coronary heart disease: results from a national representative sample *Am J Addict*. May–Jun; 20 (3): 257–63

19   Arriola L et al. (2010) Alcohol intake and the risk of coronary heart disease in the Spanish EPIC cohort study *Heart*. Jan; 96 (2): 124–30.

20   *Maclure M.* (1993) *Demonstration of deductive meta-analysis: ethanol intake and risk of myocardial infarction. Epidemiol Rev;* 15: 328–51.

21   Ronksley PE et al. (2011). Association of alcohol consumption with selected cardiovascular disease outcomes: a systematic review and meta-analysis. *British Medical Journal*, Feb 22; 342: d671

Chapter 4

1   *Diabetes Care* January 2004 vol. 27 no. suppl 1 s47

2   PR Newswire; *Transparency Market Research* "Global Diabetes Market: Drugs & Devices (2011–2016), November 1, 2011

3   Baliunas DO et al. (2009) Alcohol as a risk factor for type 2 diabetes: A systematic review and meta-analysis *Diabetes Care*. Nov; 32 (11): 2123–32.

4   Koppes LL et al. (2005) Moderate alcohol consumption lowers the risk of type 2 diabetes: a meta-analysis of prospective observational studies. *Diabetes Care*. 2005 Mar; 28 (3): 719–25

5   Reis JP et al. (2011). Lifestyle Factors and Risk for New-Onset Diabetes: a Population-Based Cohort Study *Annals of Internal Medicine*, *155*(5), 292–99.

6   Beulens JW (2012) Alcohol consumption and risk of type 2 diabetes in European men and women: influence of beverage type and body size . *J Intern Med*. 272(4):358–70.

7   Pietraszek A, Gregersen S, Hermansen K. (2010). Alcohol and type 2 diabetes. A review. *Nutr Metab Cardiovasc Dis*.; 20 (5): 366–75

8   *Drugwatch* Avandia Lawsuit, 10 Dec 2012

9   Montori VM, Isley WL, Guyatt GH (2007). Waking up from the dream of preventing diabetes with drugs. *British Medical Journal*, 334 (7599), 882.

10   Lifshitz F, Hall JG (2002). Reduction in the incidence of type II diabetes with lifestyle intervention or metformin. *J Med*, 346, 393–403.

11   Avogaro A, Tiengo A. (1993). Alcohol, glucose metabolism and diabetes. *Diabetes/metabolism reviews*, 9 (2), 129–146.

12   Konrat C et al. (2002)Alcohol intake and fasting insulin in French men and women. The D.E.S.I.R. Study. *Diabetes Metab*. 28 (2):116–23.

13   Kiechl S et al. (1996) Insulin sensitivity and regular alcohol consumption: large prospective, cross-sectional population study (Bruneck Study). *BMJ*, 313, 1040–44

14   Sierksma A et al. (2004). Effect of moderate alcohol consumption on adiponectin, tumor necrosis factor-α, and insulin sensitivity. *Diabetes Care*, 27(1), 184–89.

15   Shai I et al. (2007). Glycemic Effects of Moderate Alcohol Intake Among Patients With Type 2 Diabetes A multicenter, randomized, clinical intervention trial. *Diabetes Care*, 30(12), 3011–16.

16   Hill D, Fisher M (2010). The effect of intensive glycaemic control on cardiovascular outcomes. *Diabetes, Obesity and Metabolism*, 12(8), 641–647.

17   *New York Daily News*, 30 Jan 2013

18   Lindtner C et al. (2013). Binge drinking induces whole-body insulin resistance by impairing hypothalamic insulin action. *Science Translational Medicine*, 5(170), 170ra14.

19   Binge Drinking Increases Risk of Type 2 Diabetes by Causing Insulin Resistance. *NY (PRWEB)* 30 Jan 2013

Chapter 5

1   Källberg H (2009) Alcohol consumption is associated with decreased risk of rheumatoid arthritis; Results from two Scandinavian case-control studies *Ann Rheum Dis*. 2009 February; 68 (2): 222–27

2   Di Giuseppe D et al. (2012) Long term alcohol intake and risk of rheumatoid arthritis in women: a population based cohort study. *British Medical Journal*, 345. e4230

3   Jin Z et al. (2013) Alcohol consumption as a preventive factor for developing rheumatoid arthritis: a dose-response meta-analysis of prospective studies *Ann Rheum Dis* doi:10.1136/annrheumdis: 2013–203323

4   Maxwell JR, Gowers IR, Moore DJ, Wilson AG (2010). Alcohol consumption is inversely associated with risk and severity of rheumatoid arthritis *Oxford Rheumatology* 49 (11): et al.2146

5   Jonsson M et al. (2007) Ethanol prevents development of destructive arthritis. *Proceedings of the National Academy of Sciences*, 104(1), 258–

263.

6   Imhof A et al. (2004) Overall alcohol intake, beer, wine, and systemic markers of inflammation in western Europe: results from three MONICA samples (Augsburg, Glasgow, Lille). *European Heart Journal, 25*(23), 2092–2100.

7   Singh JA et al. (2009) Biologics for rheumatoid arthritis: an overview of Cochrane reviews. *Cochrane Database Syst Rev, 4*(4).

8   Marrone JA et al. (2012) Moderate alcohol intake lowers biochemical markers of bone turnover in postmenopausal women. *Menopause, 19*(9), 974–979.

9   Mukamal KJ et al. (2007) Alcohol consumption, bone density, and hip fracture among older adults: the cardiovascular health study *Osteoporosis International* 18, (5) 593–602.

Cawthon PM. et al (2006) Alcohol intake and its relationship with bone mineral density, falls, and fracture risk in older men *J Am Geriatr Soc.* 54 (11): 1649–57.

10   Curhan GC et al. (1996) Prospective study of beverage use and the risk of kidney stones. *American Journal of Epidemiology,* 143 (3), 240–47.

11   Curhan GC et al. (1998) Beverage use and risk for kidney stones in women. *Annals of Internal Medicine,* 128 (7), 534–40.

12   William Shakespeare *"The Tragedy of Macbeth"* Act 2, scene 3

13   Men's genital sexual arousal and alcohol intoxication: A critical re-appraisal.. *World Congress of Sexology* Havana, Cuba. March 2003

14   George WH et al. (2006) Alcohol and erectile response: the effects of high dosage in the context of demands to maximize sexual arousal. *Experimental and Clinical Psychopharmacology,* 14 (4), 461.

15   Morlet A et al. (1990) Effects of acute alcohol on penile tumescence in normal young men and dogs. *Urology,* 35 (5), 399–404.

16   Chew KK, Bremner A, Stuckey B., Earle C, Jamrozik K (2009) Alcohol Consumption and Male Erectile Dysfunction: An Unfounded Reputation for Risk? *The Journal of Sexual Medicine,* 6 (5), 1386–94.

17   Jiann BP (2010). Effect of Alcohol Consumption on the Risk of Erectile Dysfunction. *Urological Science,* 21(4), 163–68

18   Venkov CD et al. (1999) Ethanol increases endothelial nitric oxide production through modulation of nitric oxide synthase expression. *Thrombosis and Haemostasis-Stuttgart,* 81, 638–42.

19   George WH et al. (2011) Women's sexual arousal: Effects of high alcohol dosages and self-control instructions. *Hormones and behavior,* 59 (5), 730–38.

20   Glynn RJ et al. (1985) The development of benign prostatic hyperplasia. *American Journal of Epidemiology,* 121 (1), 78–90.

21   Parsons JK, Im R (2009). Alcohol consumption is associated with a decreased risk of benign prostatic hyperplasia. *The Journal of Urology*, 182 (4), 1463–68.

Chapter 6

1   Crews FT et al. (2004). Alcohol☒Induced Neurodegeneration: When, Where and Why? *Alcoholism: Clinical and Experimental Research*, 28 (2), 350–64.

2   Morris SA et al. (2010) Alcohol inhibition of neurogenesis: a mechanism of hippocampal neurodegeneration in an adolescent alcohol abuse model. *Hippocampus*, 20 (5), 596–607.

3   Gupta S, Warner J (2008) Alcohol-related dementia: a 21st-century silent epidemic? *The British Journal of Psychiatry*, 193 (5), 351–53.

4   Badsberg-Jensen G, Pakkenberg B (1993) Do alcoholics drink their neurons away? *Lancet* 342: 1201–04.

5   Harper C (1998) The neuropathology of alcohol-specific brain damage, or does alcohol damage the brain? *Journal of Neuropathology and Experimental Neurology*, 57 (2), 101–10.

6   Oscar-Berman M, Marinkovic K (2003) Alcoholism and the brain: an overview. *Alcohol Research and Health*, 27 (2), 125–33.

7   Åberg E, Hofstetter CP, Olson L, Brené S. (2005) Moderate ethanol consumption increases hippocampal cell proliferation and neurogenesis in the adult mouse. *The International Journal of Neuropsychopharmacology*, 8 (04), 557–67

8   Britton A, Singh-Manoux A, Marmot M (2004) Alcohol Consumption and Cognitive Function in the Whitehall II Study. *American Journal of Epidemiology,* 160 (3), 240–47.

9   Stephens DN, Duka T (2008) Cognitive and emotional consequences of binge drinking: role of amygdala and prefrontal cortex. *Philosophical Transactions of the Royal Society B: Biological Sciences*, 363 (1507), 3169–79.

10   Neafsey EJ, Collins MA (2011) Moderate alcohol consumption and cognitive risk. *Neuropsychiatric Disease and Treatment*, 7, 465.

11   Gupta S, Warner J (2008) Alcohol-related dementia: a 21st-century silent epidemic? *The British Journal of Psychiatry*, 193 (5), 351–53.

12   Espeland MA et al. (2005) Association between reported alcohol intake and cognition: results from the Women's Health Initiative Memory Study. *American Journal of Epidemiology*, 161 (3), 228–238.

13   Ganguli M et al. (2005) Alcohol consumption and cognitive function in late life. A longitudinal community study. *Neurology*, 65 (8), 1210–1217.

14   Weyerer S et al. (2011) Current alcohol consumption and its relationship to incident dementia: results from a 3-year follow-up study

among primary care attenders aged 75 years and older. *Age and Ageing*, 40 (4), 456–63.

15   Peters R et al. (2008) Alcohol, dementia and cognitive decline in the elderly: a systematic review. *Age and Ageing*, 37 (5), 505–12.

16   Anstey KJ, Mack HA, Cherbuin N (2009) Alcohol consumption as a risk factor for dementia and cognitive decline: meta-analysis of prospective studies. *American Journal of Geriatric Psych*, 17 (7), 542–55

17   Neafsey EJ. op.cit.

18   Truelsen T, Thudium D, Grønbæk M (2002) Amount and type of alcohol and risk of dementia. The Copenhagen City Heart Study. *Neurology*, 59 (9), 1313–19.

19   Orgogozo JM et al. (1997) Wine consumption and dementia in the elderly: a prospective community study in the Bordeaux area. *Revue Neurologique*, 153 (3), 185–92

20   Rushworth JV, Griffiths HH, Watt NT, Hooper NM (2013) Prion protein-mediated toxicity of amyloid-β oligomers requires lipid rafts and the transmembrane LRP1. *Journal of Biological Chemistry*, 288 (13): 8935–51.

21   Collins MA et al. (2010) Moderate ethanol preconditioning of rat brain cultures engenders neuroprotection against dementia-inducing neuroinflammatory proteins: possible signaling mechanisms. *Molecular Neurobiology*, 41 (2–3), 420–25.

22   den Heijer T et al. (2004) Alcohol intake in relation to brain magnetic resonance imaging findings in older persons without dementia. *The American Journal of Clinical Nutrition*, 80 (4), 992–97.

23   Pohlack ST et al. (2012) Bigger is better! Hippocampal volume and declarative memory performance in healthy young men. *Brain Structure and Function*, 1–13.

24   Solfrizzi V et al. (2007) Alcohol consumption, mild cognitive impairment, and progression to dementia. *Neurology*, 68 (21): 1790–99.

25   Xu G et al. (2009) Alcohol consumption and transition of mild cognitive impairment to dementia. *Psychiatry and Clinical Neurosciences*, 63 (1), 43–49.

Chapter 7

1   Lieber CS (1991) Perspectives: do alcohol calories count? *American Journal of Clinical Nutrition,* 54 (6), 976–82.

2   Wang L et al. (2010). Alcohol consumption, weight gain, and risk of becoming overweight in middle-aged and older women. *Archives of Internal Medicine*, 170(5), 453.

3   Tolstrup JS et al (2008) Alcohol drinking frequency in relation to

subsequent changes in waist circumference. *The American Journal of Clinical Nutrition*, (4), 957–63.

4   Wannamethee SG, Field AE, Colditz GA, Rimm EB (2004) Alcohol Intake and 8☒Year Weight Gain in Women: A Prospective Study. *Obesity Research*, 12(9), 1386–96.

5   Liu S et al. (1994) A prospective study of alcohol intake and change in body weight among US adults. *American Journal of Epidemiology*, 140 (10), 912–20.

6   Sung KC, Kim SH, Reaven GM (2007) Relationship among alcohol, body weight, and cardiovascular risk factors in 27,030 Korean men. *Diabetes Care*, 30 (10), 2690–94.

7   Cordain L, Bryan ED, Melby CL, Smith MJ (1997) Influence of moderate daily wine consumption on body weight regulation and metabolism in healthy free-living males. *Journal of the American College of Nutrition*, 16(2), 134–39

8   Westerterp-Plantenga MS, Verwegen CR (1999) The appetizing effect of an aperitif in overweight and normal-weight humans. *The American Journal of Clinical Nutrition*, 69 (2), 205–12.

9   Suter PM, Schutz Y, Jequier E (1992) The effect of ethanol on fat storage in healthy subjects *N Engl J Med.* 9; 326 (15): 983–7.

10   Jéquier, E. (1999) Alcohol intake and body weight: a paradox. *The American Journal of Clinical Nutrition*, 69 (2), 173–74.

11   Sonko BJ et al. (1994) Effect of alcohol on postmeal fat storage. *The American Journal of Clinical Nutrition*, 59 (3), 619–625.

12   Atwater WO, Snell JF (1903) Description of a bomb-calorimeter and method of its use. *Journal of the American Chemical Society*, 25 (7), 659–99.

13   Sabaté J (2003) Nut consumption and body weight. *The American journal of Clinical Nutrition*, 78 (3), 647S–650S.

14   Brehm BJ, Seeley RJ, Daniels SR, D'Alessio DA (2003) A randomized trial comparing a very low carbohydrate diet and a calorie-restricted low fat diet on body weight and cardiovascular risk factors in healthy women. *Journal of Clinical Endocrinology & Metabolism*, 88 (4), 1617–23.

15   Jéquier E (1999) op. cit.

16   Suter PM (1997) How much do alcohol calories count? *Journal of the American College of Nutrition,* 16 (2), 105–06

17   Kuhn TS (1962) "The structure of scientific revolutions". *University of Chicago Press.*

18   Aguiar AS, Da-Silva VA, Bonaventura GT (2004) Can calories from ethanol contribute to body weight preservation by malnourished rats? *Brazilian Journal of Medical and Biological Research*, 37 (6), 841–46.

19   Hackney JF, Engelman RM, Good RA (1992) Ethanol calories do

not enhance breast cancer in isocalorically fed C3H/Ou mice. *Nutrition & Cancer,* 18 (3): 245–53

20   Smith RR et al.(2009) Ethanol consumption does not promote weight gain in female mice. *Annals of Nutrition and Metabolism,* 53(3–4), 252–59.

21   Lieber CS (1991) op. cit.

Chapter 8

1   Montignac M (1986) *Dine Out & Lose Weight* [self-published]

2   Thomas DE, Elliott EJ, Baur L (2007) Low glycaemic index or low glycaemic load diets for overweight and obesity. *Cochrane Database Syst Rev,* 3 (3).

3   Hätönen KA et al. (2012) Modifying effects of alcohol on the postprandial glucose and insulin responses in healthy subjects. *The American Journal of Clinical Nutrition,* 96 (1), 44–49.

4   Tolstrup JS. Et al. (2008) Alcohol drinking frequency in relation to subsequent changes in waist circumference. *The American Journal of Clinical Nutrition,* 87 (4), 957–63.

5   Vadstrup ES, Petersen L, Sørensen TIA, Grønbaek M (2003) Waist circumference in relation to history of amount and type of alcohol: results from the Copenhagen City Heart Study. *International Journal of Obesity,* 27 (2), 238–46.

6   Dorn JM et al. (2003) Alcohol drinking patterns differentially affect central adiposity as measured by abdominal height in women and men. *Journal of Nutrition,* 133 (8), 2655–62.

7   Bobak M, Skodova Z, Marmot M (2003) Beer and obesity: a cross-sectional study. *European Journal of Clinical Nutrition,* 57 (10), 1250–53.

8   Lukasiewicz E et al. (2005) Alcohol intake in relation to body mass index and waist-to-hip ratio: the importance of type of alcoholic beverage. *Public Health nutrition,* 8 (03), 315–20.

9   Schütze M et al (2009) Beer consumption and the 'beer belly': scientific basis or common belief & quest. *European Journal of Clinical Nutrition,* 63 (9), 1143–49.

10   Bergmann MM et al. (2011) The association of lifetime alcohol use with measures of abdominal and general adiposity in a large-scale European cohort. *European Journal of Clinical Nutrition,* 65 (10), 1079–87.

11   Sayon-Orea C et al. (2011) Type of alcoholic beverage and incidence of overweight/obesity in a Mediterranean cohort: the Sun project. *Nutrition,* 27 (7), 802–08.

12   Dallongeville J et al. (1998) Influence of alcohol consumption and various beverages on waist girth and waist-to-hip ratio in a sample of

French men and women. *International Journal of Obesity*, 22 (12), 1178–83.

13   Caton SJ, Ball M, Ahern A, Hetherington MM (2004) Dose-dependent effects of alcohol on appetite and food intake. *Physiology & Behavior*, 81(1), 51–58.

14   Yeomans MR, Phillips MF (2002) Failure to reduce short-term appetite following alcohol is independent of beliefs about the presence of alcohol. *Nutritional Neuroscience*, 5 (2), 131.

15   Calissendorff J et al. (2005) Inhibitory effect of alcohol on ghrelin secretion in normal man. *European Journal of Endocrinology*, 152 (5), 743–47.

16   Caton SJ, Bate L, Hetherington MM (2007) Acute effects of an alcoholic drink on food intake: aperitif versus co-ingestion. *Physiology & Behavior*, 90 (2), 368–75.

17   Alcohol & Obesity; an overview. National Obesity Observatory/NHS Feb 2012 http://www.noo.org.uk/NOO_pub/briefing_papers

Chapter 9

1   Parry CD, Patra J, Rehm J (2011) Alcohol consumption and non☒communicable diseases: epidemiology and policy implications. *Addiction,* 106 (10), 1718–24.

2   Alcohol-related deaths in the United Kingdom 2011: http://www.ons.gov.uk/ons/dcp171778_296289.pdf

3   Rehm J et al. (2010) The relation between different dimensions of alcohol consumption and burden of disease: an overview. *Addiction,* 105 (5), 817–43.

4   Corrao G, Rubbiati L, Zambon A, Aricò S (2002).Alcohol☒attributable and alcohol☒preventable mortality in Italy A balance in 1983 and 1996. *European Journal of Public Health*, 12 (3), 214–23.

5   Gerloff A, Singer MV, Feick P (2010).Beer and its non-alcoholic compounds: role in pancreatic exocrine secretion, alcoholic pancreatitis and pancreatic carcinoma. *International Journal of Environmental Research and Public Health*, 7 (3), 1093–04.

6   Naveau S et al. (2013) Body Fat Distribution and Risk Factors for Fibrosis in Patients with Alcoholic Liver Disease. *Alcoholism: Clinical and Experimental Research* Feb; 37 (2): 332–8

7   McDonnel R, Maynard A (1985) Estimation of life years lost from alcohol-related premature death. *Alcohol and Alcoholism*, 20 (4), 435–43.

8   John U et al. (2013). Excess Mortality of Alcohol☒Dependent Individuals After 14 Years and Mortality Predictors Based on Treatment Participation and Severity of Alcohol Dependence. *Alcoholism: Clinical and Experimental Research*, 37 (*1),* 156–163.

9   Doll R, Hill AB (1956) Lung cancer and other causes of death in

relation to smoking. *British medical journal*, 2 (5001), 1071.

10   Doll R, Peto R, Hall E, Wheatley K, Gray R (1994) Mortality in relation to consumption of alcohol: 13 years' observations on male British doctors. *British Medical Journal*, 309 (6959), 911.

11   Holahan CJ et al. (2010) Late⊠Life Alcohol Consumption and 20⊠ Year Mortality, *Alcoholism: Clinical and Experimental Research*, 34 (11), 1961–71.

12   Rehm J, Sempos CT (1995) Alcohol consumption and all⊠cause mortality. *Addiction*, 90 (4), 471–80.

13   Fuchs CS et al. (1995) Alcohol consumption and mortality among women. *New England Journal of Medicine*, 332 (19), 1245–1250.

14   Grønbæk M et al. (2000) Type of alcohol consumed and mortality from all causes, coronary heart disease, and cancer. *Annals of Internal Medicine*, 133 (6), 411–19.

15   Shaper AG, Wannamethee G, Walker M (1988) Alcohol and mortality in British men: explaining the U-shaped curve. *The Lancet*, 332 (8623), 1267–73

16   Fillmore KM et al. (2007) Moderate alcohol use and reduced mortality risk: systematic error in prospective studies and new hypotheses. *Annals of Epidemiology*, 17(5), S16–S23.

17   Holahan CJ (2010) op. cit.

18   Ronksley PE et al. (2011) Association of alcohol consumption with selected cardiovascular disease outcomes: a systematic review and meta-analysis. *British Medical Journal*, *342*: d67

19   Mukamal KJ, Chiuve SE, Rimm EB (2006) Alcohol consumption and risk for coronary heart disease in men with healthy lifestyles. *Archives of Internal Medicine*, 166 (19), 2145.

20   Holman CD, English DR, Milne E, Winter MG (1996) Meta-analysis of alcohol and all-cause mortality: a validation of NHMRC recommendations.
The Medical Journal of Australia, 164 (3), 141.

21   Di Castelnuovo A t al. (2006) Alcohol dosing and total mortality in men and women: an updated meta-analysis of 34 prospective studies. *Archives of Internal Medicine*, 166 (22), 2437.

22   Schmidt W, Popham RE, Israel Y (1987) Dose⊠Specific Effects of Alcohol on the Lifespan of Mice and the Possible Relevance to Man. *British Journal of Addiction*, 82 (7), 775–88

23   Di Castelnuovo A (2006) op. cit.

Chapter 10

1   Dudley R (2000) Evolutionary origins of human alcoholism in primate frugivory. *Quarterly Review of Biology*, 3–15

2   Parlesak A et al. (2002) Gastric alcohol dehydrogenase activity in

man: influence of gender, age, alcohol consumption and smoking in a Caucasian population. *Alcohol and Alcoholism*, 37 (4), 388–93

3   Frezza M et al. (1990) High blood alcohol levels in women: the role of decreased gastric alcohol dehydrogenase activity and first-pass metabolism. *New England Journal of Medicine*, 322 (2), 95–99

4   Chrostek L, Jelski W, Szmitkowski M, Puchalski Z (2003) Gender⊠related differences in hepatic activity of alcohol dehydrogenase isoenzymes and aldehyde dehydrogenase in humans. *Journal of Clinical Laboratory Analysis*, 17 (3), 93–96.

5   Epstein EE, Fischer-Elber K, Al-Otaiba Z (2007) Women, aging, and alcohol use disorders. *Journal of Women & Aging*, 19 (1–2), 31–48.

6   McKnight D (2002) "From hunting to drinking: The devastating effects of alcohol on an Australian Aboriginal community". *Psychology Press*.

7   Mancall PC (1997) "Deadly medicine: Indians and alcohol in early America". *Cornell University Press*.

8   Ehlers, C. L., Liang, T., & Gizer, I. R. (2012). ADH and ALDH polymorphisms and alcohol dependence in Mexican and Native Americans. *The American Journal of Drug and Alcohol Abuse*, 38 (5), 389–94.

9   Ian Mortimer (2012) "The Time Traveller's Guide to Elizabethan England" The Bodley Head

10   Goedde, H. W., Agarwal, D. P., Harada, S., Rothhammer, F., Whittaker, J. O., & Lisker, R. (1986). Aldehyde dehydrogenase polymorphism in north American, south American, and Mexican Indian populations. *American journal of human genetics*, 38 (3), 395.

11   Luo HR et al. (2009) Origin and dispersal of atypical aldehyde dehydrogenase *Gene*, 435 (1), 96–103

12   Goedde HW, Harada S, Agarwal DP (1979). Racial differences in alcohol sensitivity: a new hypothesis. *Human Genetics*, 51 (3), 331–34.

13   Li D, Zhao H, Gelernter J (2012) Strong protective effect of the aldehyde dehydrogenase gene (ALDH2) 504lys (* 2) allele against alcoholism and alcohol-induced medical diseases in Asians. *Human Genetics*, 131 (5), 725–37.

14   Osier MV et al. (2002) A Global Perspective on Genetic Variation at the ADH Genes Reveals Unusual Patterns of Linkage Disequilibrium and Diversity. *American Journal of Human Genetics*, 71 (1), 84–99

15   Kendler KS, Gardner C, Dick DM (2011) Predicting alcohol consumption in adolescence from alcohol-specific and general externalizing genetic risk factors, key environmental exposures and their interaction. *Psychological Medicine*, 41 (7), 1507–1516.

16   Nurnberger J Jr., Bierut L (2007) Seeking the connections:

alcoholism and our genes. *Scientific American Magazine*, 296 (4), 46–53.

17   Nurnberger J (2007) op. cit.

18   Monzoni A et al. (2001) Genetic determinants of ethanol-induced liver damage. *Molecular Medicine,* 7 (12), 255–262

19   Nagata N et al. (2002) Assessment of a difference in ALDH2 hetero-zygotes and alcoholic liver injury. *Alcoholism, Clinical and Experimental Research,* 26 (8):11S–14S

20   Hines LM et al. (2001) Genetic variation in alcohol dehydrogenase and the beneficial effect of moderate alcohol consumption on myocardial infarction. *New England Journal of Medicine*, 344 (8), 549–55.

21   Kim SW et al. (2010) The role of acetaldehyde in human psychomotor function: a double-blind placebo-controlled crossover study. *Biological psychiatry*, 67 (9), 840–45.

Chapter 11

1   Diagnostic and Statistical Manual of Mental Disorders, Fourth Edition – Text Revision (DSMIV-TR) *American Psychiatric Association*

2   Heather N (2012) Can screening and brief intervention lead to population-level reductions in alcohol-related harm?. *Addiction Science & Clinical Practice*, 7 (1), 15.

3   *Ibid.*

4   Nurnberger J (2007) op. cit.

5   Williams SH (2005) Medications for treating alcohol dependence. *Am Fam Physician*, 72 (9), 1775–80.

6   Spanagel R, Kiefer F (2008) Drugs for relapse prevention of alcoholism: ten years of progress. *Trends in Pharmacological Sciences*, *29*(3), 109–115

7   Lötterle J, Husslein EM, Bolt J, Wirtz PM (1989) Diurnal differences in alcohol absorption. *Blutalkohol*, 26 (6), 369.

8   *The Telegraph,* 6 Jan 2010

9   Gea A et al. (2013) Alcohol intake, wine consumption and the development of depression: the PREDIMED study. *BMC Medicine*, 11 (1), 192.

10   Boden JM, Fergusson DM (2011) Alcohol and depression. *Addiction*, 106 (5), 906–14.

Chapter 12

1   Bessaoud F, Daurès JP (2008) Patterns of alcohol (especially wine) consumption and breast cancer risk: a case-control study among a population in Southern France. *Annals of Epidemiology*, 18 (6), 467–75.

2   Dennis J et al. (2010) Alcohol consumption and the risk of breast cancer among BRCA1 and BRCA2 mutation carriers. *Breast,* 19 (6), 479–83.

3   Boyd NF et al (1998) Mammographic densities and breast cancer risk. *Cancer Epidemiology Biomarkers & Prevention*, 7 (12), 1133–44.

4   Flom JD et al. (2009). Alcohol intake over the life course and mammographic density. *Breast Cancer Research and Treatment*, 117 (3), 643–51.

5   Shufelt C et al. (2012) Red versus white wine as a nutritional aromatase inhibitor in premenopausal women: A pilot study. *Journal of Women's Health*, 21 (3), 281–84.

6   Schlachterman A et al. (2008) Combined resveratrol, quercetin, and catechin treatment reduces breast tumor growth in a nude mouse model. *Translational Oncology*, 1(1), 19–27.

7   Whitsett T, Carpenter M, Lamartiniere CA (2006) Resveratrol, but not EGCG, in the diet suppresses DMBA-induced mammary cancer in rats. *Journal of Carcinogenesis*, 5 (1), 15.

8   Newcomb PA et al (2009) No Difference Between Red Wine or White Wine Consumption and Breast Cancer Risk Cancer Epidemiol Biomarkers *Prev.* 18(3): 1007–1010.

9   Pedersen A, Johansen C, Grønbæk M (2003) Relations between amount and type of alcohol and colon and rectal cancer in a Danish population based cohort study. *Gut*, 52 (6), 861–67.

10   Park JY et al. (2009) Baseline alcohol consumption, type of alcoholic beverage and risk of colorectal cancer in the European Prospective Investigation into Cancer and Nutrition-Norfolk study. *Cancer Epidemiology*, 33 (5), 347–54.

11   Han X et al. (2010) Alcohol consumption and non-Hodgkin lymphoma survival. *Journal of Cancer Survivorship*, 4 (2), 101–09.

12   Talamini R et al. (2008) The impact of tobacco smoking and alcohol drinking on survival of patients with non⊠Hodgkin lymphoma. *International Journal of Cancer*, 122 (7), 1624–29.

13   Chao C (2007) Associations between beer, wine, and liquor consumption and lung cancer risk: a meta-analysis. *Cancer Epidemiology Biomarkers & Prevention*, 16 (11), 2436–47.

14   Chao C et al. (2008) Alcoholic beverage intake and risk of lung cancer: the California Men's Health Study. *Cancer Epidemiology Biomarkers & Prevention*, 17 (10), 2692–99.

15   Barstad B et al. (2005) Intake of wine, beer and spirits and risk of gastric cancer. *European Journal of Cancer Prevention*, 14 (3), 239–43.

16   Schoonen WM et al. (2005) Alcohol consumption and risk of prostate cancer in middle⊠aged men. *International Journal of Cancer*, 113 (1), 133–140.

17   Schuurman AG, Goldbohm RA, van den Brandt PA (1999) A prospective cohort study on consumption of alcoholic beverages in

relation to prostate cancer incidence (The Netherlands). *Cancer Causes & Control*, 10 (6), 597–605.

18 Brizuela L et al. (2010) The sphingosine kinase-1 survival pathway is a molecular target for the tumor-suppressive tea and wine polyphenols in prostate cancer. *The FASEB Journal*, 24 (10), 3882–94.

19 Grønbæk M et al. (1998) Population-based cohort study of the association between alcohol intake and cancer of the upper digestive tract. *BMJ*, 317 (7162), 844–48.

20 Vioque J et al. (2008) Esophageal cancer risk by type of alcohol drinking and smoking: a case-control study in Spain. *BMC Cancer*, 8 (1), 221.

21 Kubo A et al. (2009) Alcohol types and sociodemographic characteristics as risk factors for Barrett's esophagus. *Gastroenterology*, 136 (3), 806–15.

22 Mehlig K et al. (2008) Alcoholic beverages and incidence of dementia: 34-year follow-up of the prospective population study of women in Göteborg. *American Journal of Epidemiology*, 167 (6), 684–91.

23 Truelsen T, Thudium D, Grønbæk M (2002) Amount and type of alcohol and risk of dementia The Copenhagen City Heart Study. *Neurology*, 59 (9), 1313–19.

24 Letenneur L. (2004) Risk of dementia and alcohol and wine consumption: a review of recent results. *Biological Research*, 37 (2), 189–94.

25 Luchsinger JA et al. (2004) Alcohol intake and risk of dementia. *Journal of the American Geriatrics Society*, 52 (4), 540–46.

26 Corder EH et al. (1993). Gene dose of apolipoprotein E type 4 allele and the risk of Alzheimer's disease in late onset families. *Science*, 261 (5123), 921–23.

27 Obisesan TO et al. (1998) Moderate wine consumption is associated with decreased odds of developing age-related macular degeneration in NHANES-1. *Journal of the American Geriatrics Society*, 46 (1), 1–7.

28 Mondaini N et al. (2009) Regular moderate intake of red wine is linked to a better women's sexual health. *Journal of Sexual Medicine*, 6 (10), 2772–77.

29 www.fsfiquestionnaire.com

30 Fukuhara S et al. (2011). Vardenafil and resvol synergistically enhance the nitric oxide/cyclic guanosine monophosphate pathway in corpus cavernosal smooth muscle cells and its therapeutic potential for erectile dysfunction in the streptozotocin-induced diabetic rat: preliminary findings. *Journal of Sexual Medicine,* 8 (4), 1061–71.

31 Renaud SD, de Lorgeril M (1992) Wine, alcohol, platelets, and the

French paradox for coronary heart disease. *The Lancet*, 339 (8808), 1523–26.

32   *CBS News*, "The French Paradox" November 1991

33   Estruch R et al. (2004) Different effects of red wine and gin consumption on inflammatory biomarkers of atherosclerosis: a prospective randomized crossover trial: effects of wine on inflammatory markers. *Atherosclerosis*, 175 (1), 117–23.

34   Chiva-Blanch G et al. (2012) Effects of red wine polyphenols and alcohol on glucose metabolism and the lipid profile: a randomized clinical trial. *Clinical Nutrition*, 32 (2), 200–06.

35   Estruch R et al. (2011) Moderate consumption of red wine, but not gin, decreases erythrocyte superoxide dismutase activity: a randomised cross-over trial. *Nutrition, Metabolism and Cardiovascular Diseases*, 21 (1), 46–53.

36   Sacanella E et al. (2007) Down-regulation of adhesion molecules and other inflammatory biomarkers after moderate wine consumption in healthy women: a randomized trial. *American Journal of Clinical Nutrition*, 86 (5), 1463–69.

37   Rotondo S, Di Castelnuovo A, de Gaetano G (2001) The relationship between wine consumption and cardiovascular risk: from epidemiological evidence to biological plausibility. *Italian Heart Journal*, 2 (1), 1.

38   Klatsky AL (2010) Alcohol and cardiovascular health. *Physiology & behavior*, 100 (1), 76–81.

39   Renaud SC et al. (2004) Moderate wine drinkers have lower hypertension-related mortality: a prospective cohort study in French men. *The American Journal of Clinical Nutrition*, 80 (3), 621–25.

40   Dixon JB, Dixon ME, O'Brien PE (2002) Reduced plasma homocysteine in obese red wine consumers: a potential contributor to reduced cardiovascular risk status. *European Journal of Clinical Nutrition*, 56 (7), 608–14.

41   di Giuseppe R et al. (2009) Alcohol consumption and n–3 polyunsaturated fatty acids in healthy men and women from 3 European populations *Am J Clin Nutr* 89: 354–62.

42   Curhan GC et al. (1996) Prospective study of beverage use and the risk of kidney stones. *American Journal of Epidemiology*, 143 (3), 240–47.

43   Curhan GC, Willett WC, Speizer FE, Stampfer MJ (1998) Beverage use and risk for kidney stones in women. *Annals of Internal Medicine*, 128 (7), 534–40.

44   Thomson CA et al. (2012) Alcohol consumption and body weight change in postmenopausal women: results from the Women's Health Initiative. *International Journal of Obesity*, 36 (9), 1158–64.

45   Takkouche B et al. (2002). Intake of wine, beer, and spirits and the risk of clinical common cold. *American Journal of Epidemiology*, 155 (9), 853–58.

46   305 Cohen S et al. (1993) Smoking, alcohol consumption, and susceptibility to the common cold *Am J Public Health*. 83 (9): 1277–83.

47   Grønbæk M et al. (2000) Type of alcohol consumed and mortality from all causes, coronary heart disease, and cancer. *Annals of Internal Medicine*, 133 (6), 411–19.

48   Klatsky AL et al. (2003) Wine, liquor, beer, and mortality. *American Journal of Epidemiology*, 158 (6), 585–95.

49   *Annals of Internal Medicine*, Summary for patients. 19 Sept 2000

50   German BJ, Walzem RL (2000) The health benefits of wine. *Annual Review of Nutrition,* 20, 561–93.

51   McDonald J (1986), Nutrition, A Symposium on Wine, Health and Society *Wine Institute*, Washington. D.C. 24 February

52   Paganga G, Miller N, Rice-Evans CA (1999) The polyphenolic content of fruit and vegetables and their antioxidant activities. What does a serving constitute? *Free Radical Research*, *30* (2), 153–62.

53   German JB (2000) op. cit.

54   PubMed, accessed 6 Oct 2013

55   Arranz S et al. (2012) Wine, beer, alcohol and polyphenols on cardiovascular disease and cancer. *Nutrients*, 4 (7), 759–81.

56   Jang M et al. (1997) Cancer chemopreventive activity of resveratrol, a natural product derived from grapes. *Science*, 275 (5297), 218–20.

57   Lu F et al. (2008) Resveratrol prevents estrogen-DNA adduct formation and neoplastic transformation in MCF-10F cells. *Cancer Prevention Research*, 1 (2), 135–145.

58   Chen S et al. (1998) Suppression of breast cancer cell growth with grape juice. *Pharmaceutical biology*, 36, 53–61.

59   Eng ET et al. (2003) Suppression of estrogen biosynthesis by procyanidin dimers in red wine and grape seeds. *Cancer Research*, 63 (23), 8516–8522.

60   Eng ET et al. (2002) Anti⊠Aromatase Chemicals in Red Wine. *Annals of the New York Academy of Sciences*, 963 (1), 239–46.

61   D'Archivio M et al. (2010) Bioavailability of the polyphenols: status and controversies. *International Journal of Molecular Sciences*, 11 (4), 1321–42.

62   Del Rio D, Stewart AJ, Pellegrini N (2005) A review of recent studies on malondialdehyde as toxic molecule and biological marker of oxidative stress. *Nutrition, Metabolism and Cardiovascular Diseases*, 15 (4), 316–28.

63   Gorelik S et al. (2008) The stomach as a "bioreactor": when red meat meets red wine. *Journal of Agricultural and Food Chemistry*, 56 (13), 5002–07.

64   Patel KR et al. (2013) Sulfate Metabolites Provide an Intracellular Pool for Resveratrol Generation and Induce Autophagy with Senescence

Sci Transl Med 5, 205ra133 DOI: 10.1126

65   pers.comm.

66   "Resveratrol Health Benefits: The Red Wine Myth". Online article by Francis Lichtenberger – http://www.healthfitnessexperts.com/health-benefits-resveratrol/

67   Professor David Sinclair, Harvard Medical School, reported in *AAAS News* 7 Mar 2013

68   *2nd International Conference on Resveratrol and Health*. Summary of Scientific Working Group Discussion, University of Leicester. 8 Dec 2012

69   Kwon JY et al. (2012) Piceatannol, natural polyphenolic stilbene, inhibits adipogenesis via modulation of mitotic clonal expansion and insulin receptor-dependent insulin signaling in early phase of differentiation. *Journal of Biological Chemistry*, 287 (14), 11566–78.

70   Takkouche B et al. (2002) op. cit.

71   Arranz S et al. (2012) op. cit.

72   *FASEB Journal*, 11 June 2010

73   Cordova AC, Sumpio BE (2009) Polyphenols are medicine: Is it time to prescribe red wine for our patients?. International Journal of Angiology, *18* (3), 111.

Chapter 13

1   Costanzo S et al. (2011) Wine, beer or spirit drinking in relation to fatal and non-fatal cardiovascular events: a meta-analysis. *Eur J Epidemiol.* Nov; 26 (11): 833–50

2   Mayer O (2001) population study of the influence of beer consumption on folate and homocysteine concentrations. *Eur J Clin Nutr.* Jul; 55 (7): 605–9.

3   Thrift AP et al. (2011), Lifetime Alcohol Consumption and Risk of Barrett's Esophagus *American Journal of Gastroenterology* 106, 1220–30

4   Murray LJ et al. (2002) Inverse relationship between alcohol consumption and active Helicobacter pylori infection: the Bristol Helicobacter project. *Am J Gastroenterol.* Nov; 97 (11): 2750–5.

5   Liu R et al. (2013) Alcohol Consumption, Types of Alcohol, and Parkinson's Disease. *PLoS ONE* 8(6): e66452. doi:10.1371

6   Johansen D, Friis K, Skovenborg, Grønbæk M (2006) Food buying habits of people who buy wine or beer: cross sectional study. *British Medical Journal*, 332 (7540), 519

Chapter 15

1   *Daily Mail* online, 14 Nov 2011

2   *The Times* 13 July 2013

3   *The Telegraph* 4 June 2013

4   *The Telegraph* 3 Jan 2013

5   Boniface S, Shelton N (2013) How is alcohol consumption affected if we account for under-reporting? A hypothetical scenario. *The European Journal of Public Health.*

6   Patra J et al. (2010) Alcohol consumption and the risk of morbidity and mortality for different stroke types-a systematic review and meta-analysis. *BMC Public Health*, 10 (1), 258.

7   Renaud SC et al. (2004) Moderate wine drinkers have lower hypertension-related mortality: a prospective cohort study in French men. *The American Journal of Clinical Nutrition*, 80 (3), 621–625.

8   Estruch R et al. (2011) Moderate consumption of red wine, but not gin, decreases erythrocyte superoxide dismutase activity: a randomised cross-over trial. *Nutrition, Metabolism and Cardiovascular Diseases*, 21 (1), 46–53.

9   Wannamethee SG, Shaper AG (2003) Alcohol, body weight, and weight gain in middle-aged men. *The American Journal of Clinical Nutrition*, 77 (5), 1312–17.

10   Diaz LE et al. (2002) Influence of alcohol consumption on immunological status: a review. *European Journal of Clinical Nutrition*, 56 (3), S50–S53.

11   Hackney JF (1992) op. cit.

12   Key J et al. (2006) Aug Meta-analysis of studies of alcohol and breast cancer with consideration of the methodological issues. *Cancer Causes Control* 17 (6): 759–70.

13   *WCRF/AICR Continuous Update Project Report*, October 2010. The Associations between Food, Nutrition and Physical Activity and the Risk of Colorectal Cancer.

14   Park JY et al. (2010) Alcohol intake and risk of colorectal cancer: Results from the UK Dietary Cohort Consortium. *British Journal of Cancer*, 103 (5), 747–56.

15   Midanik L (1982) The validity of self-reported alcohol consumption and alcohol problems: A literature review. *British Journal of Addiction*, 77 (4), 357–82

16   Knibbe RA, Bloomfield K (2001) Alcohol consumption estimates in surveys in Europe: comparability and sensitivity for gender differences. *Substance Abuse*, 22 (1), 23–38.

17   Rey G, Boniol M, Jougla E (2010) Estimating the number of alcohol⊠attributable deaths: methodological issues and illustration with French data for 2006. *Addiction*, 105 (6), 1018–29.

18   Northcote J, Livingston M (2011) Accuracy of self-reported drinking: observational verification of 'last occasion' drink estimates of young adults. *Alcohol and Alcoholism*, 46 (6), 709–13

19   Stockwell T et al. (2004) Under-reporting of alcohol consumption in household surveys: a comparison of quantity–frequency, graduated–frequency and recent recall. *Addiction*; 99: 1024–33

20   Truelsen T, Thudium D, Grønbæk M (2002) Amount and type of alcohol and risk of dementia The Copenhagen City Heart Study. *Neurology*, 59 (9), 1313–19.

21   Schoeller D.A (1990) How Accurate Is Self-Reported Dietary Energy Intake? *Nutrition Reviews* 48 (10) 373–79.

22   "Statistics on Alcohol: England" (2012) NHS Health and Social Care Information Centre.

23   Alcohol-related deaths in the United Kingdom 2011: http://www.ons.gov.uk/ons/dcp171778_296289.pdf

24   Naveau S et al. (2012) op.cit.

25   *The Telegraph* 17 Jun 2009

26   for example, Ellison RC. (2005) Importance of pattern of alcohol consumption. *Circulation.* Dec 20; 112 (25): 3818–9.

27   Danel T, Touitou Y (2004) Chronobiology of alcohol: from chronokinetics to alcohol-related alterations of the circadian system. *Chronobiology International*, 21 (6), 923–35.

28   Halsted CH et al.(2002) Metabolic interactions of alcohol and folate. *J Nutr* 132: 2367S–2372S.

29   Mason JB, Choi SW (2005) Effects of alcohol on folate metabolism: implications for carcingenesis *Alcohol.* Apr; 35 (3): 235–4

30   Sellers TA et al. (2001) Dietary folate intake, alcohol, and risk of breast cancer in a prospective study of postmenopausal women. *Epidemiology,* 12 (4), 420–428.

31   Zhang S et al. (1999) A prospective Study of Folate Intake and the Risk of Breast Cancer *JAMA.* 1999;281 (17): 1632–37

32   Wien TN et al.(2012) Cancer risk with folic acid supplements: a systematic review and meta-analysis. *BMJ Open,* 2 (1).

33   Chacko BK et al. (2011) Mitochondria⊠targeted ubiquinone (MitoQ) decreases ethanol⊠dependent micro and macro hepatosteatosis. *Hepatology*, 54 (1), 153–63.

34   Di Castelnuovo A et al. (2006) op. cit.

35   *Washington Post,* 2 Nov 2011

36   BBC Radio 4, *You and Yours* 4 Jan 2013.

37   *Daily Mail*, 8 August 2013

38   White IR, Altmann DR, Nanchahal K (2002) Alcohol consumption and mortality: modelling risks for men and women at different ages. *BMJ* 325 (7357), 191.

Appendix One

1   Friedenreich CM. (2011) Physical activity and breast cancer: review of the epidemiologic evidence and biologic mechanisms. *Recent Results Cancer Res.* 188: 125–39.

2   Suzuki R et al. (2005). Alcohol and postmenopausal breast cancer risk defined by estrogen and progesterone receptor status: a prospective cohort study. *Journal of the National Cancer Institute,* 97 (21), 1601–08.

3   Kent, A. (2012). Alcohol and breast cancer. *Reviews in Obstetrics and Gynecology,* 5 (1), 57.

4   Key J et al. (2006). Meta-analysis of studies of alcohol and breast cancer with consideration of the methodological issues. *Cancer Causes & Control,* 17 (6), 759–70.

5   Breast cancer risk factors; Age. *Cancer Research UK* Accessed 6 Oct 2013

6   R Curtis Ellison (2011) Effects of Alcohol on Cardiovascular Disease Risk, Preventive Cardiology:A Companion to Braunwald's Heart Disease, *Elsevier*

Appendix Two

1   Ponz de Leon M, (2010) *Intern Emerg Med*, DOI 10. 1007/s 11739–010–0487–1.

2   Di Castelnuovo A (2010) *Intern Emerg Med* DOI 10.1007/s 11739 – 010 – 0502–6.

3   Estruch R (2010) *Intern Emerg Med* DOI 10.1007/s 11739 – 010 – 0503–5.

4   Critique 029: Differing opinions on the message to the public regarding alcohol consumption 16 January 2011, Boston University School of Medicine.

5   *Ibid.*

6   *Ibid.*

7   *Ibid.*

8   *Ibid.*

9   *Ibid.*

10   *Ibid.*

11   Klatsky A.(2007) Panel Discussion V: The Message on Moderate Drinking, *Ann Epidemiol* 17: S110–S111.

12   Edited uncorrected transcripts of HC-1928-I, April 2012, HC-1936-I October 2011

13   Health Education Authority, UK. September 1996. ISBN 0752107267

Index

How many grams per drink?

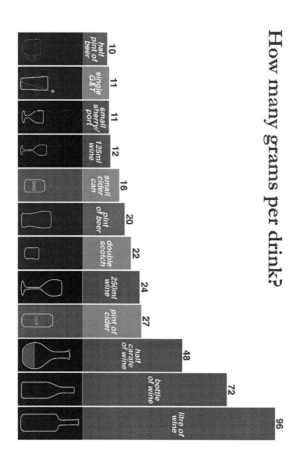

half pint of beer	10
single G&T	11
small sherry/ port	11
125ml wine	12
small cider can	16
pint of beer	20
double scotch	22
250ml wine	24
pint of cider	27
half carafe of wine	48
bottle of wine	72
litre of wine	96

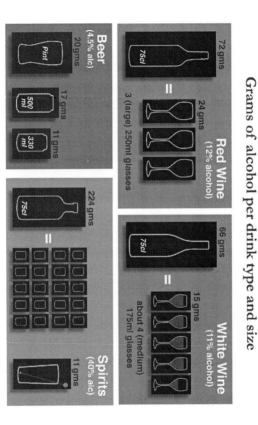

Grams of alcohol per drink type and size